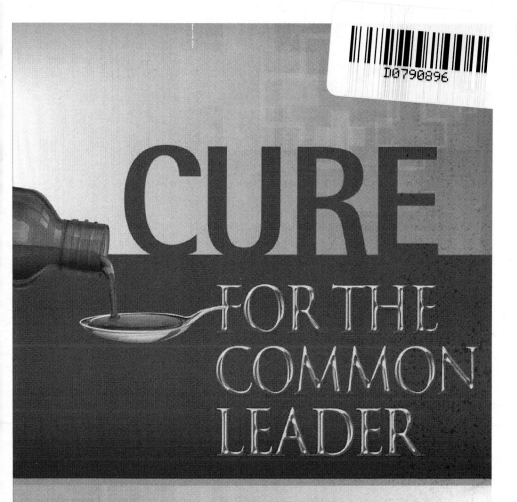

CURE
FOR THE COMMON LEADER

What Physicians & Managers
Must Do to Engage & Inspire
Healthcare Teams

Joe Mull

Cure for the Common Leader

What Physicians & Managers Must Do to Engage & Inspire Healthcare Teams

A Joe Mull Book

Copyright © 2014, Joe Mull, Ally Training & Development

Book Cover by Tracey Miller | www.TraceOfStyle.com

Publishing by Weston Lyon | www.WestonLyon.com

Edited by Lauren Cullumber

ISBN: 1502975157

EAN-13: 978-1502975157

This book is dedicated to all who work on the front lines of healthcare, for when we are sick, scared, and overwhelmed, you help us through it. Thank you for your service to us all.

About the Author

Joe Mull is President of Ally Training & Development (AllyTraining.com), which provides leadership development, management training, and staff development programs exclusively to healthcare organizations.

Prior to launching his own firm, Joe was head of Learning and Development for Physician Services at a *U.S. News and World Reports* Top 10 Hospital System, where he directed learning strategy and implementation for more than 9,000 employees at over 500 locations.

A dynamic, engaging speaker, Joe has trained more than 30,000 people over a 14-year career, turning managers into strong leaders.

He is a Certified MBTI Practitioner, has trained with the Disney Business Institute, and is in demand as a speaker and trainer on leadership and employee engagement in healthcare.

Joe holds a Masters degree in Education from Ohio University and resides in the suburbs of Pittsburgh, PA with his wife and two children.

Cure for the Common Leader

Table of Contents

Introduction

There are more than 11,000 hospitals and 550,000 outpatient ambulatory health care sites in the United States. These sites employ more than 830,000 physicians and more than 290,000 medical and health care services managers.

My job is to equip them with the leadership skills they need to navigate the people management challenges they face every day.

I've spent 14 years designing and delivering training programs. For almost ten years I've worked exclusively in healthcare. As a former head of learning and development at a U.S. News and World Reports Top 10 hospital and healthcare system, I spent thousands of hours assessing organizational and team needs, coaching managers and physicians, designing and delivering training interventions and development programs, bringing new sites online, onboarding, and helping leaders mediate team dysfunction and conflict. I've worked directly in a variety of healthcare environments, partnering with hospitals, physician practices, labs, urgent-care centers, cancer centers, family practices, and a multitude of hospital-based specialties, including anesthesiology, women's health, otolaryngology, pediatrics, and more.

It was during the course of this work that I repeatedly encountered physicians and managers thirsty for resources to help them become better leaders. Specifically, they wanted help tackling the people management challenges they faced in their role. What are people management challenges? That's the term I use to describe all the non-technical problems leaders face when building and leading teams. People management challenges are the interpersonal and performance management issues leaders of every stripe face in almost every industry.

These problems show up every day and demand the time, energy, and attention of leaders in ways that are hard to quantify. Conflict, poor employee performance, time and attendance issues, lack of effort, insubordination, and gossip are all people management challenges.

Among these many issues, however, there is one in particular that has loomed large over others. It's the question I was asked the most in the early years of my career providing leadership and management training to healthcare personnel:

"How do I motivate my team?"

Year after year I was repeatedly asked for insight into how leaders spark team members to try harder, give their all, and showcase enthusiasm for their work. As a result, I began seeking answers grounded in research and psychology. I spent the next several years examining the body of evidence on employee engagement and motivation and integrating my findings into the leadership training I design and deliver. What I discovered, and what much of the social science research on motivation suggests, is that the answer to the question "How do I motivate my team?" is just two words:

You don't.

Motivation isn't something you do to someone. It's something employees experience when the conditions are right. Leaders cannot reach inside their individual contributors and flip a switch that ignites a drive to perform. What they must do is install those conditions that meet the complex emotional and professional needs of employees to trigger motivation in each person. Creating work environments that lead to engaged, motivated healthcare employees therefore requires leaders to possess 1) insight into what conditions employees must experience to be engaged, and 2) leadership skills related to communication, feedback, and cultivating purpose (among others) to actively create those conditions. When leaders develop this unique blend of knowledge and skill, they become equipped to influence the psychological commitment employees have to their work.

That is what I hope to accomplish with this book.

Training physicians and managers on how to engage healthcare teams is the entirety of my professional focus and the foundation of the company I founded, Ally Training & Development. We endeavor to give physicians and managers this unique combination of knowledge and skill through interactive, evidence-based training. Nowadays I travel the country speaking at conferences and delivering training on-site on what physicians and managers must do to create engaging workplaces for healthcare teams. When physicians and managers become the kind of boss for whom others want to work, engagement increases, motivation is present, and people management challenges recede.

This book is about fostering employee engagement in healthcare. In the pages ahead, I will translate the latest research on leadership, engagement, and motivation into SEVEN actions physicians and managers must take to engage and inspire healthcare teams. These actions are based on data, conclusions, and recommendations from established, reputable sources. These sources include the National Center for Healthcare Leadership, the Accreditation Council for Graduate Medical Education, and Gallup, the world's leading researcher on employee engagement. (A complete list of references appears at the end of the book). They are also based on my 14 years of experience training and coaching leaders.

Each chapter is packed with dozens of tips, tricks, ideas, suggestions, strategies, and exercises to help you implement and sustain each of the seven actions. Whether you currently work as a physician, practice manager, unit director, chief nursing officer or you aspire to one of these roles; there is something for you in this book. Likewise, if you hire, train, support, supervise, or partner with physicians or managers, I'm confident this book will provide insight and information that will serve you well.

For some of you, this book will challenge your belief system about what your job truly is. It will require you to become a leader of *people*. To invest your time, energy, and focus on the individuals that make up your team, what they need to be successful, and how you, as their boss, work to provide that every day. Be cautious about dismissing recommendations you perceive to be less important. You are naturally going to assign value to some recommendations over others based on your own bias. Remember that just because something isn't important to you doesn't mean it's not important to someone else.

The research is clear. The shortest path to patient satisfaction, lower turnover, and higher productivity in healthcare is a leader on-site who knows how to get their teams firing on all cylinders. I'm going to teach you how to do just that.

Let's get started.

Chapter 1

The Case For Engagement

A variety of factors influence the effort and enthusiasm employees bring to their jobs. Before we can explore the actions leaders must take to bring out the best in people, we have to first examine and understand these influences. At the center of this examination is a term I have referenced already and that you've likely heard before.

Employee engagement.

It's a shame that in recent years the concept of employee engagement – a critical one for managers and leaders at all levels to understand – has achieved a kind of buzzword status. Many in number are the consultants, companies, and authors who claim expertise in engagement without full knowledge of what it is, how it is measured, and how it can be influenced.

DEFINING ENGAGEMENT

While many reputable organizations have been examining employee engagement in recent years, none has done more work on the subject over a greater period of time than Gallup. For more than 30 years, Gallup has studied employee engagement in the workplace. They've partnered with thousands of companies, in every imaginable industry, to examine just what leads to the highest levels of employee performance and contribution. To date, they've surveyed more than 25 million employees in over 160 countries. Gallup defines employee engagement as "the degree to which *employees are invested in and enthusiastic about their work and thus act in a way that furthers the interests of the organization.*"

Put another way, employee engagement is the psychological and emotional commitment individuals have to their work that leads them to *care* and *try*. And if you've been in any kind of front-line healthcare leadership role for any amount of time, you know that these things make all the difference in the world to how successfully employees serve patients, their families, and teammates.

Satisfaction ≠ Engagement

Pop quiz: When employees are happy, satisfied, and like coming to work, that means they are engaged, right?

Bzzzt. Nope. Wrong.

Engagement and job satisfaction are not the same thing. After years of investing time and resources to measure job satisfaction, companies across all industries are finally getting wise to the notion that there is limited correlation between job satisfaction and high levels of workplace performance. Why? Quite simply, it is this: there are many employees who are wholly satisfied to remain unchallenged at work every day, going through the motions, doing the minimum, and collecting a paycheck.

You've worked alongside such individuals at one point or another in your career, I'm sure.

Happiness and satisfaction relate to engagement, but alone are insufficient to create it. While an engaged employee almost certainly experiences some level of job satisfaction, a person experiencing job satisfaction isn't necessarily engaged. That person may enjoy coming to work most days, but they don't display the psychological and emotional commitment to the job that moves the organization forward. Understanding this difference, then, forces us to acknowledge something you have probably long known:

Some employees are more valuable than others.

Superstars, Sleepwalkers, and Lifesuckers

Who are your superstars at work? The folks who show up every day and give their all. They take initiative, problem-solve, serve patients to the fullest extent they can, and do so without the need to be prompted by leadership. These are the people you can't live without, the ones you would clone if you could. They are, to use the aforementioned definition, fully invested in and enthusiastic about the work they do. These are your ENGAGED employees. They care, and they try. They act in such a way that furthers the interests of the organization, teammates, and patients. Research suggests just 30% of the U.S. workforce falls into this category.

Analysis of engagement data suggests there are two other kinds of employees on your team: Not Engaged and Actively Disengaged. These folks cost you every day that they are allowed to occupy space in your organization.

Employees who are Not Engaged don't always appear to do harm. They are the sleepwalkers and daydreamers in your enterprise. They show up, go through the motions, and leave. They rarely do more than what is required or expected. They are uninvested. While you are busy giving your all, they are clock-watching and making their grocery list. More than half (52%) of the U.S. workforce is not engaged at work. Yikes!

Your Actively Disengaged employees, it will come as no surprise, pose a significant threat to your team and patients. Actively Disengaged employees act out their unhappiness at work. They give voice to negativity and undermine what others are trying to achieve. They are short with patients, battle with those around them, say, "That's not my job," and serve as a detrimental influence on team culture and performance. In a word, they are *toxic*. They are the lifesuckers in any organization. Roughly 18% of employees are Actively Disengaged.

IMPACT AND OUTCOMES

One of the behaviors most commonly associated with engagement is *discretionary effort*. What is discretionary effort? It's the difference in the level of effort one is capable of bringing to an activity or a task and the effort required only to get by or make do. Discretionary effort only comes from engaged employees and is but one of the numerous ways engagement manifests itself in employee performance. There are others – initiative, problem solving, energy level, and continuous improvement among them.

If employee engagement only revealed itself in this way, in the performance of individual contributors, that alone might motivate some to strive for and attend to its cultivation. But engagement doesn't just show itself in the day-to-day actions of employees. Many of the key performance indicators healthcare systems and teams use to gauge organizational performance are metrics that reflect engagement. These include turnover, productivity, absenteeism, retention, patient satisfaction, and profitability, to name a few. Engaged, Not Engaged, and Actively Disengaged employees have a quantifiable impact on an organization at almost every level.

Engaged employees create new and repeat visits, drive innovation and growth, expend the most energy at work, demonstrate higher levels of creativity and productivity, and contribute to higher revenues. They make fewer errors, miss fewer days, and almost exclusively generate new and repeat customers.

Employees who are Not Engaged are less attentive to customers, less productive, create more waste, and expend less effort. Because they are essentially "checked out," they display little or no concern for customers, productivity, profitability, waste, safety, mission and purpose of the team, or developing new business.

Actively Disengaged employees are responsible for more complaints, theft, accidents, and quality defects than other employees. They monopolize managers' time, have increased time and attendance issues, and have a direct, negative influence on retention, turnover, productivity, and reputation.

In their 2013 *State of the American Workplace Report*, Gallup confirmed the connection (well-established in other research) between employee engagement and nine performance outcomes: customer ratings, profitability, productivity, turnover, safety incidents, theft, absenteeism, patient safety incidences, and quality defects. They also found that:

- The top 25% of teams have nearly 50% fewer accidents and have 41% fewer quality defects.

- Actively disengaged employees cost the U.S. between $450 and $550 billion each year in lost productivity.

- Engaged employees have significantly higher productivity, profitability, and customer ratings, less turnover and absenteeism, and fewer safety incidents.

- Actively Disengaged employees are much more likely to steal from their companies. In fact, almost all theft in an organization comes from this group.

- When patients and families encounter engaged teams, it increases the likelihood that they will be forgiving in the face of mistakes or subpar service.

Engagement impacts performance across all layers of an organization. When high levels of engagement are present, it leads to a culture where members of the team are willing to do "whatever it takes," which directly impacts patient satisfaction, new and repeat traffic, reputation, and revenue.

If you're reading this book, then I assume those are things you care a great deal about. The next question, then, is at the core of what this book is about: How do you create engaged employees?

THE PATH TO ENGAGEMENT

There is compelling evidence to suggest that several conditions must be present to cultivate engagement. Leading researchers in employee engagement – companies like Gallup, AonHewitt, BlessingWhite, and The Ken Blanchard Companies – all describe the circumstances that create engagement with their own unique vocabulary, but a perusal of the body of research makes clear that certain elements are at the core of fostering engagement. Employees are likely to be engaged when they experience:

- Opportunities to learn, grow, and advance

- Alignment of their talents and skills to their job

- Making a difference and doing work that matters (what we'll call *purpose*)

- Opportunities to form meaningful relationships with teammates and leaders

- Having the information, materials, and equipment necessary to do the job

- Their opinions are solicited and considered

- Recognition

When employees go to work and experience most or all of these conditions, they thrive. They are more likely to stay, perform, and positively impact the overall business. These are the conditions that create the psychological and emotional commitment that leads to discretionary effort.

Look closely at this list, and one thing becomes abundantly clear: engagement is a local phenomenon between employees and the leaders they see every day.

The Boss Matters

Time for another pop quiz. What is the single most influential factor in employee engagement?

A. Pay and benefits

B. Nature of the work

C. Relationship with manager

D. Opportunities to advance

While many instinctively choose A, that's not the answer. Compensation certainly plays a part in affecting motivation and engagement, but not nearly to the degree most believe. Social science research on what drives people at work reveals that salary, benefits, and other compensatory factors influence motivation only to the degree that they are *fair and adequate*. If an employee believes their compensation is unfair - that others on the team or in their field receive higher levels of compensation - engagement CAN be impacted, even if all other conditions listed above are present. However, once an employee believes they are fairly compensated, pay and benefits no longer influence motivation. This is a key distinction to understand. Compensation's impact on engagement is limited, unless employees perceive it to be unfair or inadequate. In those cases, it can become a cause of disengagement.

So what's the answer to our quiz? While employees' levels of engagement are certainly impacted by the nature of their work and by opportunities to advance, it's the relationship with one's manager that most impacts employee engagement. Research suggests that the quality of the local workplace manager, and his or her ability to meet a complex set of emotional and professional needs, is the single most influential factor in engagement. In fact, 75% of people leaving a job indicate that their manager is part or all of the reason.

People don't quit their jobs. They quit their bosses.

An employee's direct supervisor has a profound amount of influence over their work experience every single day. If the boss believes that employees should simply show up, do their job, know their place, and be thankful they get to come back tomorrow, they are failing to meet the emotional and professional needs of the individual. This antiquated, command-and-control thinking leads to Not Engaged and Actively Disengaged employees who ultimately harm the brand or simply leave. However, if the boss installs and maintains conditions for engagement, he or she meets the emotional and professional needs of the individual. This is how the boss fosters engagement.

What's critical to recognize, though, is this: The boss is really the *only* one who can foster engagement. Take a moment to revisit that list of conditions that lead to engagement. One by one, ask yourself: *How does an employee experience this condition? Where does it come from? Who provides that to them?* It quickly becomes apparent that an employee's direct supervisor is the only person with the necessary blend of power and opportunity to cultivate engagement for each employee.

And this is where it gets tricky for healthcare. Because our employees don't have just one boss. In most cases, they have many.

Who's The Boss?

Ask your front desk person who is in charge of the practice overall. What will she say? Ask her who her boss is. Does she give the same answer?

In many healthcare settings employees interact with two levels of supervisory authority: the operational leaders charged with their day-to-day supervision, and physicians. The office manager, unit director, nurse coordinator, or practice manager oversees the day-to-day operations of the site and the duties of team members. These managers often hire, train, and supervise the employee. They coordinate the employee's schedule, answer their questions, and serve as the primary liaison between employee and employer. Physicians, on the other hand, possess a different kind of power. In most healthcare environments, but especially in out-patient settings, the employee experiences the physician as the ultimate authority and decision maker. Employees know that the manager often has to answer to or take orders from the physicians. Physicians set the tone for what happens at a site, how people interact, and the overall culture of the environment. This is why BOTH physicians AND managers must work to cultivate engagement. One leader doing so without the other limits the potential for engagement. That is not to say that if you are reading this book and work alongside a manager or physician who has NO interest in attending to engagement that you should give up. You alone can still have a significant impact for your direct reports. However, that impact becomes magnified greatly when both levels of leadership put forth the effort.

The problem in healthcare, unfortunately, is that many teams roll-up to managers with underdeveloped "soft skills" and physicians unaware of or unprepared for the key people management role they need to fill.

Healthcare is like many other industries in that we select, promote, and rely on underdeveloped managers. When someone is installed as a manager they are often selected based on clinical knowledge, operational experience, or technical expertise. Indeed, many healthcare executives will tell you plainly they seek out this kind of background *first* when searching for management personnel.

But once that manager is selected, steps into the role, and begins going about the business of managing and leading others, they figure out quickly that many of the problems they face every day are not of a clinical, operational, or technical nature: they're people problems that require the ability to communicate, negotiate, mediate, delegate, and evaluate. This is not a problem exclusive to healthcare. It's long been a management problem across most fields. Many managers ultimately come to the realization that the skill set that brought them to their role fails to aid them fully in succeeding in it.

For many physicians, the problem is greater. It's not that their people management skills are underdeveloped. It's that they have not been given the chance to build them at all, or even told that such skills are necessary for success. In 2012, the Accreditation Council for Graduate Medical Education (ACGME) admitted in their Leadership Development Curriculum for Chief Residents in Medicine that there is *"a significant void in the training and education of today's young physician leaders"* as it relates to leadership development. ACGME advocates for physicians to develop several leadership competencies related to people management, including listening skills, teambuilding, trust-building, and consensus-building. In 2011, the Center for Creative Leadership made a similar case in their white paper *Addressing the Leadership Gap in Healthcare.* After analyzing leadership effectiveness data from tens of thousands of people working in healthcare, they identified the top priority for leadership development in the healthcare sector as *"the abil-*

ity to lead employees and work in teams," strongly encouraging leaders at all levels to *"develop a more participative management style, improve their ability to build relationships and lead teams, and learn to deal more effectively with problem employees."*

From What to How

We have reached a unique crossroads in healthcare. The challenges faced by providers are more complex than ever before. Patients and families are in distress, confused, cynical, and vulnerable. The interactions we ask employees to execute daily – and the myriad emotions that accompany them – require that physicians and managers embrace their role as leaders of people with complex professional needs who must experience certain conditions in the workplace in order to succeed. Indeed, the success of any healthcare team depends on it.

The research on what employees must experience to become fully invested is clear. The chapters that follow identify the seven actions you must take to create an engaging environment and bring out the best in your people. They are in no particular order, as all are crucial components of fostering engagement.

Chapter 2
You Must Manage Individually

Think of the best boss you've ever had. What made him or her great to work for? What qualities or characteristics made them a strong, effective leader?

While the answers you came up with describe the person you had in mind, they also identify what you *needed* from that person in that time and at that place. Think about that for a moment. Let's say that the best boss you ever had was great to work for because she was approachable, supportive, and she challenged you. These answers tell us a lot about what you needed from her. As an employee you needed to be able to go to her, needed her support in the course of your work, and needed her to push you along the way to maximize your performance. If we spent a little more time on this subject I bet you would be able to identify specific behaviors she used to make you feel comfortable, supported, and challenged. The best boss you ever worked for was a good boss not because she did *those* specific things. It's because she understood that *you* needed those things and worked to provide them. Put another way: your boss met you where you were at.

There is data to support that this approach for most healthcare personnel is sorely needed. Gallup found that service workers – a category that includes most customer-facing jobs – saw the only drop in engagement levels, down three points from 32% in 2009 to 29% in 2012. These are your front-desk workers, schedulers, medical assistants, housekeeping and dietary personnel, transporters, etc. Gallup argues strongly for leaders to engage individually with these team members. Consider this from their 2013 report on engagement in the U.S. workforce:

Employees are profoundly different from one another. Factors such as age, generation, gender, education level, and tenure, for instance, all relate to engagement. Leaders encounter people with different talents, skills, and experiences whom they need to manage individually.

As we established, engaging and motivating people to higher levels of performance is about creating the conditions necessary for people to thrive, but these conditions are different from person to person. Physicians and managers must work to understand each direct report as an individual so they can then position that employee for success. This is managing individually.

In this chapter, we'll explore several actionable ways that supervisors at all levels must manage individually. They include meeting one-on-one with personnel, aligning employee strengths to the job role, providing regular feedback and coaching, and facilitating ongoing growth and development. These behaviors in particular go a long way in nurturing engagement at an individual level because they tap into what research suggests is the most powerful driver of workplace performance: intrinsic motivation.

UNDERSTANDING MOTIVATION

Across the social sciences the collective understanding of what motivates us has undergone a profound transformation. For almost 100 years behaviorists believed that all human action was motivated by external rewards, sometimes called extrinsic motivators. These are the rewards and consequences of any environment. If there is a reward for doing the behavior, or a consequence for not doing it, the prevailing thought was that human beings would be thusly motivated.

Whether you realize it or not, you probably use the prospect of a benefit or the threat of a penalty to motivate behavior daily. If you have kids at home it sounds something like this:

> *"You have to eat all your vegetables before you can have dessert."*

> *"If you clean up all of your toys I'll let you watch a cartoon before bed."*

> *"If you jump off that couch one more time, you're going to time-out!"*

At work, it probably sounds like this:

> *"If you show up late again I'll have to write you up."*

> *"Anyone that agrees to take on additional overnight shifts will be awarded the higher pay rate for those hours worked."*

> *"The patient satisfaction training modules are mandatory. Failure to complete them will disqualify providers from merit increases."*

Without question, external rewards motivate. But the motivation comes from "have to." The employee has to change their behavior to get the reward or to avoid the penalty. Relying only on the presence of external motivators makes it unlikely that they ever make the shift from "have to" to "want to."

Unless their leader taps into *intrinsic* motivation.

In the middle of the 20th century, researchers began examining another driver of human behavior: intrinsic (a.k.a. internal) motivation. If extrinsic motivation is "have to," intrinsic motivation is "want to."

Think about activities you enjoy doing. Do you have any hobbies? Do you play an instrument? Knit? Play golf? Think about your reasons for spending time, effort, and resources on these interests. There is, in all likelihood, no external reward for doing them. You are probably not golfing because you are trying to qualify for the PGA tour and launch a career as a golfer. If you play an instrument, I'd bet it's for many reasons, but not because you aspire to be a professional symphony musician. The motivation to devote time, attention, and effort to various hobbies, interests, and leisure activities comes from the inherent enjoyment of the activity. There is something about them you find fulfilling, joyful, and challenging. The opportunity to achieve at whatever activity or subject interests us unleashes your creativity and the human need to progress and accomplish.

In such cases, your behavior is *intrinsically* motivated.

What research has uncovered is that leaders who tap into intrinsic motivation get higher levels of effort and commitment from staff, and that effort is sustained over longer periods of time. When employees get the opportunity to do work that aligns with their interests and talents, that strikes just the right balance of challenge and ability, and that is connected to a larger purpose that matters to them, they will *want to* exert effort. Where intrinsic motivation is present, leaders rarely have to resort to "have to."

Tapping Into Intrinsic Motivation

In his exhaustively researched and wildly popular book *Drive: The Surprising Truth About What Motivates Us,* Daniel Pink argues that intrinsic motivation comes from having *autonomy* over work, being appropriately *challenged* by the work, and believing that the work has *purpose*. When all three of these elements are present, there's a greater chance employees will "want to" give maximum effort.

Additionally, this higher level of effort is sustainable over a longer period of time. Let's look at each of these elements.

Autonomy means choice. It means acting with independence. It means having ownership of and responsibility for important work. Pink asserts that the degree to which employees have autonomy over task, time, technique, and team correlates to their level of intrinsic motivation. While it can be challenging to increase autonomy in healthcare, which relies heavily on systems, processes, protocols, and schedules, it is not impossible. Physicians and managers who want to elevate the psychological commitment employees have to their work should identify ways to endow team members with more autonomy. Many of the strategies in this book are recommended because they directly or indirectly generate autonomy for individual contributors.

Challenge occurs when the duties and responsibilities of the job are in balance with the ability and interests of the employee. When employees are asked to take on work beyond the scope of their capabilities it can produce frustration, anxiety, and be detrimental to confidence. When given work that isn't challenging enough, employees may experience boredom, feelings of worthlessness, and even exhaustion. When the appropriate level of challenge is present, employees describe getting "lost" in their work. Challenge is defined not by the destination, but by progress. When workers at any level experience continual challenge that leads to continual growth, there are likely to be higher levels of engagement and motivation.

Purpose may be the most important element needed to tap into intrinsic motivation. When employees believe their work makes a difference it satisfies a basic human need to *matter*. In too many organizations, employees do not have a line of sight between what they do every day and the difference it makes. Physicians and managers must regularly feed a sense of purpose. They must rally their people to a cause greater than self, a cause that matters to the individual. This is done not through singular grandiose gestures, but via an ongoing stream of conversations, reminders, stories, and recognition that highlight contributions and difference making. I have devoted an entire chapter to this topic later in the book. It's that important.

So how do managers and physicians provide autonomy, challenge, and purpose? In one way or another, most every action suggested in this book contributes to one or several of these elements. It can be argued, however, that the most important delivery vehicle for these elements is one-on-one time between leaders and direct reports.

MEET ONE-ON-ONE WITH EMPLOYEES

One-on-one meetings are the lifeblood of employee engagement. This time is when leaders facilitate much of what is advocated for in this book. The behaviors you will be encouraged to use - coaching, feedback, strengths-based management, exploring interests, goal-setting, stretch assignments, professional development - all require one-on-one time to occur. If you aren't currently setting aside time to meet with direct reports, you are forfeiting the single most powerful engagement tool in your toolkit for getting the most out of people.

In a 2013 study by Training magazine, in partnership with renowned leadership group The Ken Blanchard Companies, employees across multiple industries said they wished they were meeting more frequently with their boss. An overwhelming 89% of employees want to meet at least monthly with their manager. Among those, almost half want to meet weekly. Yes, weekly. With regard to the length of these meetings, most employees (65%) said they want to meet for 30-60 minutes at a time.

Who and When

As noted in our first chapter, healthcare is unique in that employees essentially have two bosses, their front-line manager, and the physicians in their practice. For this reason, it's beneficial for each to hold one-on-one meetings in some form. The nature of their unique roles, however, will place a greater responsibility for one-on-ones with managers.

The availability of physicians to meet individually with team members obviously is limited. By and large, the front-line manager should schedule and facilitate these meetings with regularity. Physicians should still plan to connect with individual employees in this way, as a matter of strategy. I encourage physicians to ensure that employees get to sit down with one of their docs at least twice a year. The nature of these conversations will be similar to those the manager facilitates.

This does not have to be a cumbersome or time-consuming responsibility for physicians. In a practice with five physicians and 15 employees, each doctor can take on the responsibility for meeting once every six months with three employees for 30 minutes each. That amounts to three hours over the course of a year. The return on investment for this miniscule time commitment cannot be overstated. Leaders vote on what's most important to them by how they spend their time. When physicians prioritize time to connect directly with individual employees, even just a few times a year, it sends a powerful message.

How often should managers meet with direct reports? There's no singularly established guideline. I advise supervisors of the following, based on my experience working with leaders over the years:

- If you have a large team (more than 15 direct reports) meet once a month for 20-30 minutes with each employee.

- If you have a small team (less than 15) meet twice a month for 30 minutes with each employee.

I know what you're thinking. "Joe, seriously, I don't have time. Are you *kidding me*? How could I possibly fit that in?" Let me debunk this objection with some grade school math.

Let's say you work 40 hours per week. I know, I know...don't laugh. Many of you reading this book work well over 40 hours a week on a regular basis. I get that. But for the sake of this illustration, let's go with the potential minimum: 40 hours per week in a 4-week month. Here's what meeting twice a month for 30 minutes at a time looks like with seven direct reports:

40 hours per week X 4 weeks per month =   160 hours available
7 half hour meetings X 2 times per month =   7   hours   used
Time remaining each month: 153 hours

Over the course of a month, you would spend just over 4% of your time in one-on-one meetings. For the impact they can have, the cost here is minimal.

What if you have a larger team? Using the same time parameters, this is what meeting once a month with 18 direct reports looks like:

40 hours per week X 4 weeks per month =   160 hours
18 half hour meetings once per month =   9 hours
Time remaining each month: 151 hours

Here again, the effort is not terribly expensive spread out over a month. In this example, the manager is spending less than 6% of their time in one-on-one meetings.

In the event you are a manager with a high number of direct reports- 30, 40, 50+, then I strongly encourage you to examine the reporting structure of your team. Are there others along the chain of command empowered with management responsibilities? Delegate supervision responsibilities for some staff directly to them. It will reduce the strain on you and ensures employees get more attention from a supervisor with the capacity to serve them.

I can't stress enough how important it is to make time for these meetings. A significant portion of the advice, counsel, and actionable strategies in this book depend on you having ongoing one-on-one meetings with your staff. If you only take one action in the aftermath of reading this book, then this should be it. Set aside time regularly to meet individually. It's critical to your success.

MEETING CONTENT

The frequency of one-on-one meetings isn't the only dynamic to explore. What occurs during these meetings is equally important to consider. This is not project-update time. While you may do that briefly in the first few minutes, commit to making this time about the employee.

Progress toward goals, getting performance feedback, assistance with problem solving, and processing through conflict with a co-worker are the topics research suggests employees most want to talk about with their boss.

Not sure what to talk about? Ask. Sixty-nine percent of employees indicate they want to set the agenda in one-on-one meetings with their boss. In fact, allowing them to do so is an example of providing autonomy. Let employees know early on in the process that this is time set aside for them. Express your desire to check in and connect. Let them know you value their input, ideas, and concerns. You may not use the fully allotted time with each employee, and that's okay. Install the structure for these meetings and make it a part of the culture of your site, and over time a unique dialogue will unfold with each individual employee. Along the way, use this time to attend to many of the practices, topics, and questions advocated for in this book. To help get you started, see the Resource Box in this chapter for a list of 14 open-ended questions that can serve as conversation starters in one-on-one meetings. Whether you are a physician or manager, these questions can be a springboard to impactful meetings with individual contributors.

14 Conversation Starters for One-on-One Meetings

The primary vehicle you will use to manage individually is one-on-one time with your direct reports. Research suggests that, used correctly, this time plays a big role in performance, engagement, and motivation. Here are 14 open-ended conversation starters you can use to explore employee engagement:

1. What elements of your job energize you? Why?

2. At work do you have the opportunity to do what you do best every day? Why or why not?

3. What aspect of your work do you think is most worthy of recognition or praise?

4. What do we do well?

5. What can we improve on?

6. Do you feel valued as a person at work? Why or why not?

7. What would you like to learn more about?

8. What are your professional aspirations?

9. How can I aid you on your career path?

10. How do you think your work impacts the organization as a whole?

11. How would you describe the quality of the work produced by our team?

12. What types of training or development opportunities would interest you in the weeks and months to come?

13. What do you need that you are not getting?

14. What would make your job easier? More fulfilling?

Go slow. Don't try to cover all 14 at once. Pick one or two questions to focus on in a single meeting and don't be afraid to ask other open-ended (i.e. not Yes/No) questions. Also, be sure that you give your full time and attention to your employee in a private, comfortable location. Whenever possible, avoid typing, texting, or answering your phone. It can send a damaging message to employees about where they rank on your priorities list. For 12 additional questions for engaging one-on-ones, visit CureForTheCommonLeader.com and download the free *Cure for the Common Leader* Resource Kit.

FOCUS ON STRENGTHS

A key engagement strategy supported by research, and one that cultivates autonomy and challenge for employees, is aligning job duties with the specific strengths and talents possessed by the employee.

The 30% of Americans who are fully engaged in their work report that they have the chance to "do what they do best" every day. This means they get to do work that capitalizes on their skills, talents, and interests. Managers who work to understand these unique characteristics within each employee are taking a Strengths Based Management (SBM) approach, a strategy that research suggests is integral to employee engagement. More than half (52%) of Americans who use their strengths for three hours a day or less report feeling stressed. Conversely, the more hours per day that employees use their strengths, the more likely they are to report having higher levels of energy, happiness, interest, and fulfillment at work. Here again, Gallup's findings support this approach:

> *Among employees whose supervisors focused on their strengths, active disengagement fell dramatically to 1%. What's more, nearly two-thirds (61%) of these employees were engaged, twice the average (30%) of U.S workers nationwide. This suggests that if every organization in America trained their managers to focus on employees' strengths, the U.S. could easily double the number of engaged employees in the workplace with this one simple shift in approach.*

SBM means working to understand the strengths of people and positioning them to use their strengths as often as possible in their day-to-day work. In management we spend a lot of time doing the opposite: working to help people understand and improve their weaknesses. Problem areas are often the focus of feedback, performance reviews, development discussions, etc. SBM shifts this paradigm from one of becoming average in many things to excelling in a few areas.

This does not mean that you isolate employees from the parts of their job they find challenging or less appealing. When employees have daily opportunities to apply their strengths and talents, it creates a fulfilling work experience. It is clear to the employee that they are contributing, and they develop an emotional connection to their work, organization, teammates, and patients. That connection is where the inclination to give full effort comes from. And when circumstances call for the employee to take on challenging respon-sibilities or handle situations outside of their comfort zone, they are confident and invested enough to do so willingly. Focusing on strengths doesn't remove challenges for the employee...it positions them to navigate them more successfully.

Leaders can help employees identify strengths by drawing out tal-ents, knowledge, and skills. This can be done through discussion and observation. During your next round of one-on-one conversa-tions with employees ask them these questions: *Do you get to do what you do best every day? Why or why not? What aspects of your work are most satisfying? What would you like to do more of?* Let their answers and the subsequent conversation be a springboard to strengths-based management.

You will also identify strengths through observation. What kinds of abilities does the employee exhibit? Do they naturally take charge in groups or at meetings? Are they drawn to certain kinds of pro-jects or work assignments? In what areas are they a quick study, learning and applying faster than most? By tuning into what your employees do well, you may end up identifying something in some-one of which they weren't even aware.

Once you identify strengths, collaboratively with the employee and through observation, it is important to guide the employee through the process of describing them. Do not assume that employees are aware of their strengths. Instead, help them explore and articulate what they do well and what their strengths mean for them in the workplace. Only after this has taken place can the employee begin identifying opportunities to apply their strengths at work. Along the way, help coworkers learn and understand each other's strengths and how their talents complement those of others on the team.

What Makes Them Tick?

Another effective way to understand the unique skills and talents of those around you is to utilize an evidence-based assessment instrument. I use several in my work, but I am partial to the Myers-Briggs Type Indicator (MBTI), which I use extensively for leadership and team development. The MBTI is a personality assessment that helps users sort and identify naturally occurring preferences for the ways they get and focus their energy, take in information, make decisions, and orient their day-to-day lives. While many assessments are research-based or research supported, the MBTI is the only personality assessment that is research validated. This is my favorite tool due to the "aha moments" it creates for users as well as the richness of the dialogue that can occur once it is introduced. This does not mean that MBTI is the only choice. I encourage all leaders to use a research supported instrument based on sound psychological principles. Do a little bit of homework to find the one that's the best fit for your goals, needs, and time constraints. Exposing individuals and teams to new and powerful insights into what makes them tick can lead to increased awareness and changes in behavior.

When physicians and managers identify the ways employees most naturally think, feel, and behave, and build on talents to create strengths, it propels growth and fosters engagement. This approach also sends a message to employees that their employer cares about them as a person and encourages them to make the most of their strengths. The result is increased discretionary effort, a higher work ethic, and more enthusiasm and commitment day in and day out.

It's Worth It

It takes time and effort to understand the unique interests, talents, skills, strengths, and perspectives of each employee and to know how to leverage them in the interest of the employee's success. But the return on investment should eschew any hesitation you have to committing to this kind of collaboration. Managing individually – tapping into intrinsic motivation, spending one-on-one time with employees, and identifying their strengths and aligning their job accordingly – sets employees up for success. When you meet people where they are at you inspire loyalty, earn trust, are kept in the loop, and get maximum effort from those on your team.

WHAT PHYSICIANS AND MANAGERS MUST DO TO MANAGE INDIVIDUALLY

Action Items Summary:

- Foster autonomy, challenge, and purpose for each individual.

- Set-up recurring one-on-one meetings with direct reports.

- Ensure physicians also meet periodically with individuals, at least once every six months.

- For large teams, delegate supervision responsibilities to empowered downstream managers to ensure reach and effectiveness.

- Allow employees to set the agenda at one-on-one meetings.

- Use open-ended questions that explore employee goals, contributions, concerns, and ideas.

- Identify the talents and strengths of individual contributors.

- Find ways for employees to increase the use of their talents and strengths in their jobs.

- Introduce a reputable assessment instrument to give team members insight into themselves and others (and a vocabulary for communicating about differences).

Chapter 3

You Must Show Interest In And Care About The Person Inside The Employee

"So the blonde guy and the skinny girl both seem to be working out ok for us…"

Mary, the Practice Administrator, just shook her head. "What makes you say that?"

The physician, an experienced and accomplished practitioner in his specialty, replied, "Nothing in particular. It just seems like they're doing a good job out front."

"It's funny that you say that," Mary said. "Because they're both counting the days until they can transfer out of here."

"Why?!" the physician asked, clearly surprised.

"Well, for one thing, they've been here three months, and you don't even know their names."

• • • •

This story was shared with me by an attendee at a day-long leadership workshop I led for practice managers on engaging healthcare teams. Mary went on to describe the two front-desk workers feeling invisible, unappreciated, and unimportant. She described an environment where the physicians' interactions with personnel were brusque and impersonal. According to her, the physician described above wasn't the only person in the large practice who had neglected to engage the two new front desk workers. The docs, Mary stated, had "warm body syndrome." They gave the impression that each person was but a replaceable part of the machine.

The opening chapter of this book highlighted one of the more stunning statistics that studies on retention, turnover, and employee engagement continue to validate: 75% of people who voluntarily leave a position indicate that their boss is part or all of the reason why. That's *three out of every four*.

An employee's relationship with their on-site workplace manager is the single most influential factor in employee engagement. Not only because that person is largely responsible for training and developing the employee, but also because the tone set by the boss – via action and interaction - permeates every element of the employee experience. From Gallup's research:

> *Great managers engage their teams on several levels. First, they display genuine care and concern for their people. By building strong, trusting relationships with their staff, they can engender an open and positive work atmosphere in which employees feel supported and engaged.*

Healthcare employees go to work each day with more than one person in the boss role: their operational supervisor *and* physicians. While each fill differing roles, both hold power in the day-to-day life cycle of the employee's work experience. This is why both physicians and managers must work to cultivate meaningful relationships with team members. To neglect this dynamic is to cripple any prospect the team has of reaching its fullest potential.

Most leaders eventually learn that power and influence comes from relationships, not titles. Some learn this quickly. For others, it takes years. But somewhere along the path of trying to motivate and lead others they figure out that success as a leader depends entirely on their ability to form and maintain authentic relationships with those around them. That's what this chapter is about: building the kinds of relationships that contribute to engagement.

SWEAT THE SMALL STUFF

Physicians and managers have a lot of professional relationships to manage. Patients and families, colleagues, business partners, and staff are but a few. The best leaders develop credibility, cultivate influence, and engender goodwill by taking it upon themselves to learn everything they can about the people that surround them. They endeavor to learn and use names. They make a point of recalling details about others from previous interactions. Their words and body language show genuine interest in people and sensitivity to their needs. They display warmth, approachability, and work to put people at ease through dialogue and collegiality.

The National Center for Healthcare Leadership advocates for these behaviors as part of its Leadership Competency Model. They advise physicians to display *Interpersonal Understanding* to account for the increasing complexity and depth of others in a cross-cultural society. They specify that a healthcare leader who displays this competency:

> *Takes time to get to know people beyond superficial or job related information. Genuinely seeks to understand people as individuals and their points of view. Uses insights gained from the knowledge of others to know "where they are coming from" or why they act in certain ways. Makes or sustains informal contacts with others that extend beyond formal work relationships. Is approachable and able to engage in "small talk" and informal conversations. Maintains friendly relations and rapport with work*

*contacts. Finds things that one has in common with associ-
ates and uses them to build friendly relations.*

For some, these behaviors come naturally. For others, they are
barely present. The unique differences in personality, social comfort, and professional demeanor among managers and physicians
alike mean that some will have to work harder than others to be
attentive to this dynamic. Regardless of your capacity for this kind
of interaction, there are several behaviors all leaders should embrace to demonstrate authentic caring for personnel.

Know Your People

Building a genuine relationship with employees starts with simply
interacting with them with authentic interest and caring. This can
(and should) occur as part of the day-to-day exchanges leaders have
with team members. Displaying an awareness of the names of employees' spouses and children, where they went on vacation, or
what college their youngest will be attending in the fall, are just a
few of the details that demonstrate genuine interest in the person.

The caveat here, of course, is that not all employees want to self-
disclose information about their personal lives. I'm not advocating
for physicians and managers to suddenly launch a full investigation
into the intimate details of employees' lives. I am simply acknowledging that, while many employees participate comfortably in personal dialogue, others will maintain boundaries in this area. It's up
to the physician and manager to utilize polite, genuine, but most
importantly, *unintrusive* dialogue that demonstrates a sincere interest in the employee as a person, but that does not create discomfort
for that person. This is the difference between being perceived as
warm and being perceived as nosey.

Building and fostering authentic relationships with team members
also means respecting that sometimes life happens. For all of us,

things occur in our personal lives that we may have a hard time shaking off in the workplace. Expecting every employee to be at 100% every single day and to check everything they might be dealing with at the door is, at best, naïve and at worst, cold and dictatorial. People are human beings. Kids get sick. Family pets die unexpectedly. Relationships end. Demonstrate just a modicum of compassion and caring when your team members encounter life in this way, and they likely will not forget it. In some cases the compassion you demonstrate will drive the employee to reach for the resilience necessary to remain focused on the job.

Celebrate Your People

Another simple way to show interest and caring is to celebrate work anniversaries and birthdays. These are formal, once-a-year chances to acknowledge the value an employee brings to the team and the organizational affection for their continued presence and contribution. Too often though, leaders fail to do this with the sincerity and specificity needed to make it effective. Take, for example, an accounting firm that decided to acknowledge employee work anniversaries by having a small plant delivered to each employee by a local florist. On the day of their annual work anniversary, the employee arrived to work to find a plant on their desk along with a small card congratulating them on their anniversary.

In concept, it sounds like a nice gesture, doesn't it? Unfortunately, the effort backfired. Because when the employee's manager arrived to work that morning and saw the employee with their plant, they would respond like so:

"Oh, is it your anniversary today?! Well, happy anniversary!"

While the plant was a nice gift for the employee, there was nothing about the interaction that communicated genuine appreciation or affection for the *person*. In fact the interaction described above sends an opposing message: I don't care enough to remember your anniversary without prompting. At the very least, the manager above missed an easy opportunity to celebrate that employee. How could she have done that? Imagine if that employee arrived at their cubicle on the morning of their work anniversary and, instead of finding the same plant that everyone else got, instead found a card with this written inside:

Kathleen -

> *Four years ago today you joined our team, and we've truly benefited from your presence. Your outstanding customer service, "can do" attitude, and positive, warm demeanor are invaluable to all of us. I probably don't say it enough, but please know: I'm so glad you work here. Happy anniversary.*

> *~Jane*

Which gesture communicates value and impact to the employee? Which gesture taps into feelings of worth? Without question, the card achieves this where the plant does not. What that employee experiences is a powerful, personal sentiment. Knowing that the boss took time to get a card, sit down, and write out thoughts that have occurred in their head about what the employee brings to the team is powerful stuff.

(It's also a lot cheaper than sending flowers.)

As noted above, some will be better in this area than others. One of the best managers I ever worked with - Juanita deftly managed ten clinics, 42 docs, and over 180 staff - knew she was not strong in this area. She admitted to me that, early in her career, she saw no reason to engage in small talk with staff, acknowledge birthdays, or tolerate life stress entering employees' workplaces. "I felt that way for years, but it's just not practical" she now says. "I realized I wasn't creating the kind of environment people want to work in every day."

It was actually a Myers-Briggs Type Indicator workshop that opened her eyes. "I learned that because those kinds of interactions didn't come naturally to me, I avoided them. Once I acknowledged that they were an important part of giving people what they need from me as a leader, I had to figure out how to show up in that way from time to time."

What did she do?

"I delegated it," she told me. "I asked my office managers for help, since I rotate through multiple sites. Now they know to give me a heads up if something is going on with someone. If someone is going through something, or it's their birthday or they just think someone would benefit from a quick check-in from me, they let me know so I can act. It has made a huge difference in how I perceive team members AND how they perceive me."

Juanita genuinely cares about the person inside the employee. So she created a system to ensure she would be able to demonstrate that caring at appropriate times.

BE FUTURE FOCUSED

One thing that has always struck me about what it takes to foster employee engagement is the many parallels the path to engagement shares with Maslow's Hierarchy of Needs. A staple of developmental psychology, Maslow's Hierarchy outlines stages of human development that, when present and experienced, lead to the formation of a mature, healthy adult. Maslow theorized that foundationally human beings need certain physiological and environmental needs met. Thereafter is the need to belong, be respected, and develop confidence. Maturity culminates with self-actualization: the realization of a person's full potential via creativity, problem-solving, and more. (*"What a man can be, he must be." –* A. Maslow)

The conditions for fostering engaged employees follow a strikingly similar developmental path. Foundationally, employees need certain conditions to be present to do the job. Among these conditions are the necessary materials and equipment for the job and a clear understanding of what the job is. Following these, employees need to experience that someone at work cares about them as a person. They need the opportunity to form sophisticated relationships with co-workers, and they need to believe their work has value and impact. Ultimately and eventually, the employee needs opportunities to evolve in the job role- to learn and grow and progress. This is professional self-actualization, and it is why showing interest in and caring about the person inside of the employee means actively demonstrating a commitment to the employee's professional development.

Know Where They Want To Go And Help Them Get There
Most employees want to learn and grow. It's often up to their leader to facilitate that process, in partnership with the employee.

Knowing the future goals and aspirations of an employee is critical to engagement. Take the time to ask employees about their goals. Ask them where they want to be in a year, or in five. Ask them to describe where they want their career to go or what kinds of professional opportunities they'd like to pursue down the line. Conduct periodic "Stay Interviews" (see the Resource Box in this chapter). If the employee is unable to articulate goals, help draw them out. Employees without goals are like airplanes without flight plans.

They are traveling without a destination and will eventually run out of gas.

Once you have a clearer idea of their long-term desires, offer to help direct reports make progress toward their goals in whatever way you can. Write them down and review them periodically during one-on-one meetings.

Another strategy for developing others is to identify, assign, and debrief stretch assignments. A stretch assignment is a project or task given to an employee that is beyond their current knowledge or skill level, or that they have not done before. It is designed to challenge them in new ways or expose them to new skills or areas of responsibility. Stretch assignments may include managing a volunteer or intern, coordinating a new hire's onboarding and training, mentoring a junior staff member, improving a process, or leading a meeting or project group.

Strong leaders also actively seek out and share learning and development opportunities with their personnel. Identify training courses, conferences, workshops, or professional associations that align with the goals and aspirations expressed by each employee. Carve out the necessary resources (read: time and money) to support employee participation in these events. And don't just forward these kinds of opportunities via email. Actively bring them up in conversation and share your reasons for thinking a particular event or organization would be to their benefit.

Yet another strategy to develop others is to give employees a chance to write a self-review once a year. It is impossible for you, their boss, to see, recall, or document much of what your employees contribute. Not because you don't care or aren't invested. It's because you are human. You are busy and deal daily with many things that require attention. Thus, the self-review can fill in the space between what you as a supervisor can account for and what the employee sees as significant. Tell your staff that you want them to highlight what they accomplished and what they are proud of. Ask them to self-identify areas for improvement and explore steps toward career advancement. You do not need to set up a complicated process to do this, either. Take whatever evaluation your employer asks you to fill out on your direct reports and give them a blank copy. Invite them to fill it out on themselves and explain why you want them to do it. Once you receive this document, incorporate their language into your annual review document.

What if your employee states plainly that they don't have any goals? What if he or she is perfectly content to stay where they are at and do the job they are currently doing for the foreseeable future? What if they are unable to identify a single thing they are interested in learning about, improving, or pursuing? Answer: that's ok. Not everyone on your team is going to have the same amount of drive, and that's fine, as long as their contributions and performance are positive. My advice, when working with this kind of employee, is to spend your time focusing on Strengths-Based Management: aligning their talents and strengths to their job role. Find out what parts of the job they find most energizing and do what you can to position them to do that *more*. It just might spark additional interests or goals down the line.

Interest And Caring Produce A Return On Investment
Ultimately, this book focuses on what it takes to get your healthcare team firing on all cylinders. I can't stress enough how important it is for you as a leader to spend time with personnel throughout your healthcare organization interacting, asking, listening, and learning. It is in these acts that the people you work with begin to put forth discretionary effort. By seeking to know and understand, you demonstrate a commitment to them that lays the groundwork for

3 Tips For Showing Interest In And Caring About Each Employee

Use Reminders to Celebrate/Recognize. Most smartphones give you the power to schedule reminders. That is to say, you can tell your phone to remind you at a time or in a place to do something. Is a large project concluding in a week or two? Set-up a reminder to stop by a contributor's office, send the VP an email, or check in and thank each member of the team. Make this a part of your planning process for projects or whenever you prep for the week or month ahead. Does one of your direct reports have a birthday or work anniversary coming up? Schedule a reminder to pick up a card or use the location services feature to prompt you the next time you're in Starbucks to pick up a gift card. Combine a bit of effort with a bit of technology and suddenly you've mastered the art of attending to "the little things."

Do Stay Interviews. You've probably heard of Exit Interviews, the set of questions asked when an employee departs a position or employer. The goal is to understand the reasons people leave in an effort to reduce turnover. A Stay Interview acts much in the same way, but is far more proactive. It asks questions to better understand what would cause an employee to leave, thus bringing clarity to how to get them to stay. For a free copy of a Stay Interview you can use during one-on-one time, download the *Cure for the Common Leader* Resource Kit at CureForTheCommonLeader.com.

Respect Work/Life Boundaries. Be judicious about calling or texting employees away from the office or bringing workplace issues to them on scheduled days off. Set hard boundaries and build your practice so that it can function when individual contributors are away. If you are so reliant on a single person that they can't be out of touch with the site for a few days of vacation, then it is time to examine the division of responsibility and the quality of cross-training that is (or is not) taking place at your site.

a powerful relationship that is fulfilling and beneficial for everyone involved.

As many healthcare providers are being asked to do more with less, teams face numerous challenges, including fewer colleagues to help, higher volumes, and challenging patient populations. Showing interest in and caring about the person inside the employee buys you relationship capital that results in more resilience from team members in the face of these challenges. Put another way: your people will care about everything if they believe *you* care about *them*. And in those times when you need to deliver a firm message or unpleasant news to your team, that relationship capital cuts down on discord and grousing.

Remember: employees need to believe that their leaders care about them beyond the tasks and responsibilities of their job role. Be a boss who demonstrates genuine interest in and affection for each employee as a person, and you've taken critical steps to creating an atmosphere and culture that engages employees and retains talent.

WHAT PHYSICIANS AND MANAGERS MUST DO TO SHOW INTEREST AND CARING

Action Items Summary:
- Prioritize building a relationship with each employee.
- Learn and use names.
- Recall and use details from previous interactions in future conversation.
- Show genuine interest in people and sensitivity to their needs.

- Engage in informal ("small talk") conversations.

- Make eye contact, smile, and use body language that demonstrates active listening.

- Be mindful of employees' willingness to self-disclose. Watch for subtle signs of discomfort and adjust your interaction accordingly.

- Remember that life happens. Be kind and accommodating whenever possible when employees are in distress.

- Set reminders for birthdays, anniversaries, etc. Acknowledge these events in personal ways.

- Help fellow leaders know when an employee is under stress for reasons unrelated to work. This isn't a license to gossip. It's about building a culture of understanding and support.

- Use Stay Interviews, stretch assignments, self-reviews, and development opportunities to help employees progress and grow.

Chapter 4

You Must Regularly Ask For The Ideas, Opinions, And Challenges Of Each Employee

The Center for Creative Leadership is a top-ranked, nonprofit educational institution focused exclusively on leadership education and research. In 2011 the CCL published a revised edition of *Addressing the Leadership Gap in Healthcare*, a wide-ranging white paper summarizing leadership effectiveness data from nearly 35,000 people working in the field.

The key finding of the CCL study was that the top priority for leadership development in the healthcare sector should be to "improve the ability to lead employees and work in teams." They specifically advocate for a more participative management style and improving physicians' and managers' ability to build relationships with team members. From the white paper:

> *Managers who value participative management encourage others to share ideas, information, reactions, and perspectives- and they listen. They communicate well, keeping others informed, involving others in change, and paying attention to multiple perspectives. They try to understand what other people think before making judgments or decisions.*

The CCL isn't the only high-profile organization arguing for attention to this kind of leadership behavior in healthcare settings. The Accreditation Council for Graduate Medical Education (ACGME), the private professional organization responsible for the accreditation of over 9,200 residency education programs, highlights the need to seek out and hear from staff. In their *Leadership Develop-*

ment Curriculum for Chief Residents in Medicine they identify personal leadership skills "considered essential for the effective physician leader to be competent and successful within health care systems." Among these vital skills is the ability to solicit, hear, and act on input from personnel:

> *True listening involves hearing, understanding, and putting the information in context. Effective physician leaders must listen to the needs, ideas, concerns, and feedback of their staff and team members in order to identify opportunities, delegate to appropriate team members, address concerns and doubts, process feedback, and communicate in ways that are relevant to others.*

Here again Gallup's findings on engagement reflect the need to interface with staff in this way. On teams where employees are mined for ideas and input, engagement is higher. Among the 30% of the U.S. workforce who are actively engaged in their work, an overwhelming majority report that at work their opinions "seem to count."

What's key for physicians and managers to recognize is that staff level contributors will possess insight into things leaders do not or cannot see. They have a unique, informed perspective to offer, one that can contribute to better decisions and solutions for the site. What's more important to note, however, is that when employees are asked for their perspective or assessment, they experience being valued for more than just the tasks and responsibilities of their day-to-day work. They become a contributing member of the enterprise, accountable to its performance and married to its success. This is why drawing out and shining a light on employees' perspective leads to higher levels of commitment and engagement.

This chapter explores a variety of ways to do just that.

ORGANIZE OPPORTUNITIES FOR INPUT

Many leaders genuinely want to hear from their personnel. However, constant demands on their time and attention mean that weeks and even months can pass without this dialogue taking place. Despite having the best intentions, they fail to draw out employee insight because they did not intentionally plan to do so. While some employees will voluntarily give voice to their ideas, opinions, and concerns (some do this all day long), many will not share their perspective until asked. To create the conditions that lead to higher levels of engagement, you must plan to solicit feedback from team members. One powerful way to ensure this dialogue happens periodically is to plan and hold a staff retreat.

Retreat!

When planned and executed thoughtfully, an annual team retreat can be a powerful tool. It demonstrates to participants your commitment to understanding and meeting team needs and incorporating the perspectives of everyone into the operation and culture of the practice or unit. Retreats can also enhance discourse - often helping focus on mission, issues, strategy, or growth.

As someone who regularly builds and facilitates retreats for teams, I can tell you there is no "right" kind of retreat that works best. While retreats can certainly be grand affairs that take teams away from work to unique places, they can also be simple gatherings held in the conference room down the hall. They can be a week long, a day or two, or a few hours in a day. They can be filled with exercises, activities, presentations, teambuilding, and any number of eccentric components, or they can simply be a discussion - of what is working, what is not, and how to improve. What your retreat looks like and what happens there are entirely up to you and will likely be based on your budget and what you can logistically pull off. What's most important when it comes to retreat planning is to identify your goals. What do you want to accomplish at the retreat?

How will you get there? How will you know you met your objectives? Take time to answer these questions as part of the planning process to ensure your retreat is focused and purposeful.

If you need assistance planning a retreat, there are likely a variety of trainers, coaches, and consultants in your area who can help construct an interactive, purposeful, compelling staff retreat experience. Many will help lead the event as well. The expense of using external services will likely produce a return on investment that far exceeds the initial cost for these services. For more about staff retreats, see the Resource Box in this chapter.

Interactive Retreat Ideas

I'm a big fan of staff retreats. I strongly believe every team should do some kind of organized whole-staff gathering once a year. While the focus of this chapter is gathering and applying the unique perspectives of individual contributors, that's not the only thing for which a staff retreat can be used. Consider the following ideas as well.

Do a personality assessment. Giving team members a chance to understand "why I am the way I am," and to see how others are wired, can improve the performance of people, teams, and organizations. The increased awareness this brings can result in shifts in behavior, style, and approach. As discussed in the previous chapter, an assessment like the Myers-Briggs Type Indicator (MBTI) can enhance how team members make decisions, manage conflict, form and maintain relationships, communicate, and manage stress. The end goal is knowledge of how to flex one's style to be more successful as a member of the team. When held as part of a retreat they also provide a chance for team members to become aware of the unique strengths and styles of their colleagues.

Do a SWOT analysis. A SWOT analysis is a formal, structured approach to exploring organizational Strengths, Weaknesses, Opportunities, and Threats. Simply handout a 4 quadrant grid to your team and break them into small groups. Ask them to brainstorm in each area and report their ideas afterwards. Once you've captured the responses of the group, summarize an overall list for each quadrant. Use this info to set goals or divide the team into subgroups to work further on identified areas of need. Spread that work out over a period of time to ensure ongoing attention to challenges and changes.

Do a QPI analysis or exercise. As a former colleague of mine was fond of saying, "Sometimes it's the people, and sometimes it's the process." Quality and Process Improvement (QPI) work involves looking at the structure and processes that exist in a work environment, evaluating how they impact performance and workflow, and testing changes for improvement. There are numerous methodologies you can use (ex. Lean, Six Sigma, etc.), but working with a quality improvement professional is key. Invite a qualified process improvement specialist to help your team identify a simple, specific process for examination and refinement. Involving the whole team will accelerate change, implementation, and buy-in.

Whatever you elect to do, make it interactive, draw out the opinions of the team, and tap into the creativity of all in attendance. Find ways to infuse appropriate fun into your retreat as it often breaks down the tension that builds up between team members over time (as well as between the team and management). For a free copy of my Retreat Planning Guide for Physicians and Managers, download the Resource Kit at CureForTheCommonLeader.com.

Job Shadowing

Another formal way to ensure you gain exposure to the ideas, opinions, and challenges of team members is to set aside time once or twice a year for job shadowing. A job shadow is simply sitting with or following a member of your team for a period of time to better understand the work they do and the challenges they face. Instead of having a general impression of their work, or preconceived notions of what personnel in their role do all day, you get a chance to see it first-hand. The most successful leaders are well versed in the nuanced challenges employees face in their roles. How can you advocate for and serve your team members if you only have a passing understanding of their jobs?

If you elect to schedule job shadowing, make sure you have a focused conversation with the employee ahead of time about what you are doing and, most importantly, why. Let them know it's not performance-related, nor is it evaluative. Being clear that your primary goal is to better understand the complexities and challenges they face will help reduce (but admittedly not eliminate) some of the anxiety they will have about being observed.

Hold A Town Hall

Many political figures use town hall meetings, informal gatherings that allow attendees to voice opinions and ask questions, to stay in touch with their constituents. This approach has also become popular among CEOs and Executive leaders at organizations of all types. A town hall-style gathering can draw out the ideas and opinions of team members leaders otherwise might never get the chance to hear. Consider setting aside a one to two hour block of time, once a quarter, to lead this exercise. Be prepared with a few general questions:

- *What do we do well?*

- *What has to change?*

- *What's broken and in need of fixing?*

- *What isn't broken yet but will be down the road?*

- *If you were in charge, what would you do differently?*

Set a few basic ground rules up front to ensure that no ideas are held back or criticized. Don't be afraid of silence...and there will be silence early on. If there is little in the way of active participation, be prepared to share an update, tell a story, or identify a particular challenge facing the organization or team. Follow it up with some of the open-ended questions above to spark dialogue. Doing this exercise regularly installs it as a part of the culture of the team. The members of that team experience a regularly occurring, formal, structured opportunity to be heard. This can increase the perception among members that leadership actively seeks out and genuinely cares about the perspective of each individual. Such town hall forums assign value to team members' ideas and opinions and allow them to be heard, both of which are critical components of employee engagement. This approach can be used by any level of management and is especially helpful for managers with multiple sites, and for physicians with limited opportunities to interface with all team members regularly.

USE ROUTINE INTERACTION TO LISTEN AND LEARN

Not long ago, I was interviewed for a magazine article on effectively recruiting and hiring office managers for physician practices. The author and I explored the challenges they face in their roles, the skills needed to be successful in the position, and how to identify those skills during the interview process. In the course of that interview she asked, "What level of education should be required for an office manager in a healthcare setting?"

"Heck if I know," I said.

I went on to tell her that many of the best office managers I have encountered had no degree or formal training for the role. These were men and women (but overwhelmingly women) who worked their way up over several years, doing virtually every job and task in a practice setting. They worked the front desk and interfaced with patients. They learned the various scheduling and EMR software packages because they were forced to use them daily. They roomed patients, sent and received lab results, managed the inbox, participated in accreditation and auditing, trained staff, managed schedules, and so much more. They were scrappy. And by the time they ascended to a management position, it was second nature for them to spend much of their time working alongside the team, day in and day out.

Make Time To Work In The Trenches

For many of the managers reading this book, this is a familiar story. If not by choice, then by necessity. The reality of working in healthcare means being confronted daily with understaffed clinics, overbooked schedules, and navigating the problems posed daily by call-offs, employees on leave, terminations, and processes that place an emphasis on balancing quality with volume. Many of you are out there alongside your teams already because it's the only way the work can possibly get done. I know it's exhausting. I know it means the stuff you are *supposed* to be doing as a manager gets left for times when you'd rather not be working (see: early mornings, nighttime, weekends). It may not bring you a great deal of comfort, but it has a powerful impact on your team's perceptions of you as a leader. Perhaps most importantly, it positions you to hear and understand the ideas, needs, challenges, and concerns of the team. Physicians work side-by-side with team members every day. Managers, on the other hand, may have to be intentional about making this happen.

If you spend most of your working time behind a desk, in an office, on a computer, and bouncing from meeting to meeting, then it becomes easy for the people you serve to adopt a mindset that "she doesn't understand what we face everyday." But if you can carve out time to work directly with your teams, the results are dramatic.

You don't have to have clinical skills or training to work in the trenches with your teams and be of value to them in this way. As long as you are willing to do everything. Adopt the philosophy that nothing is beneath you. Not stocking rooms or pushing carts or wiping toilets. I know great managers who clean out the lounge refrigerator once a month because it's the least appealing task among the team. That stuff gets noticed.

Identify ways to ease the load on your team. If you don't know how to do something, learn. Ask members of your team to teach you. When you show up as a student, as a willing receiver of information, you subtly model the kind of approach you want them to take each day. As a manager there will be times when you will need to correct them, guide them, or teach them to do something differently. Their receptiveness to that feedback will be considerably higher if you have demonstrated an openness to feedback and improvement.

Being front and center on a regular basis provides you with daily opportunities to solicit and understand what individuals face in their day-to-day work, what frustrates and concerns them, and what they need to be successful. Also, remember that visibility breeds trust. The manager who comes of out of their office to say "Hey, I see we had quite a crush today, thanks for of all your hard work," will never generate the kind of loyalty among their staff as the manager who worked through it with them.

Ask the Right Questions
Working side-by-side with your team provides an almost endless number of opportunities to draw out the ideas, opinions, and challenges of team members. It is also important to ask the right ques-

tions during huddles, meetings, and other team gatherings, to integrate their perspective into the fabric of what happens at the site.

Examine the ways you share information with team members. Do you hold morning huddles? Do you post info in the staff lounge? Do you disseminate updates via email? Each of these touch points is an opportunity to solicit team member insight.

Get into the habit of using open-ended questions to draw out staff feedback as part of whatever vehicle or forum you use to share information and update your team. At team huddles ask, *"What concerns do you have about what was just shared?"* In emails, invite your audience to respond with suggestions by stating, *"I'd like to hear your ideas on the best way to...solve this problem, implement this change, etc."* You might even consider setting up an old fashioned "suggestion box" in the staff lounge to capture ideas and concerns as they strike members of the team.

Time Is The Investment
Many of the strategies suggested in this chapter require physicians and managers to use a precious and often limited resource: time. In fact, one of the biggest arguments I hear about attending to employee engagement is simply, "I don't have time." This is a false argument.

If you consider the amount of time you spend tackling performance issues, picking up the slack for unengaged or underperforming staff, or replacing those who have departed, it becomes clear that I'm not asking you to find new time as much as I'm suggesting that there is potential for an exchange of how you spend time. When you install the conditions suggested in this book, there is a high likelihood that many of the people management challenges you currently devote time to will begin to recede. And which would you rather spend your time on? Approaches that lead to engaged teams, or ongoing people management challenges that require reaction and drain your energy?

The good news is that the time needed to execute many of the ideas put forth in this chapter is negligible. An annual staff retreat, quarterly town hall forums, and the use of open-ended questions at meetings and during already-occurring interactions require a small fraction of time during the course of the year and some intentionality in planning. That's all. Setting up a two-way open dialogue with your team creates one of the key workplace conditions that lead to engagement, which pays dividends well beyond the annual time investment.

WHAT PHYSICIANS AND MANAGERS MUST DO TO DRAW OUT THE IDEAS, OPINIONS, AND CHALLENGES OF EMPLOYEES

Action Items Summary:

- Hold an annual retreat to mine staff for ideas and input.

- Spend time shadowing employees to understand the nuances of their job and the unique challenges they face.

- Hold occasional town-hall style meetings to allow employees to ask questions, voice opinions, and stay in touch with leadership.

- Work in the trenches alongside employees to ensure exposure to challenges and needs.

- Be willing to do anything. Take on unappealing tasks or ask, "How can I help?"

- Ask employees to teach you something and help you develop additional knowledge and skills.

- After sharing info and updates, draw out feedback with open-ended questions like: "What concerns do you have about what was just shared?"

Chapter 5

You Must Foster Group Cohesion And Team Spirit

Gallup's research suggests having strong relationships with colleagues at work, and even having a "best friend" at work, is critical for employee engagement and retention. On the flip side, environments where conflict and disrespect run rampant have higher rates of turnover, errors, and accidents and have lower patient satisfaction scores.

Research on adult learning theory suggests that adults retain 10% of what they read, 15% of what they hear, and 85% of what they experience. What happens at work every day becomes learned behavior. If bullying, negative attitudes, and minimal effort are present and tolerated, they become the norm. But if people get along, communicate appropriately, and treat each other with courtesy and respect, then *that* becomes the norm. It becomes the culture of the team.

In their book *Change the Culture, Change the Game (2011)* Roger Connors and Tom Smith define culture as simply "how we do things around here." High-functioning, engaged teams have leaders who foster group cohesion and team spirit because of how profoundly it impacts workplace culture. They create opportunities for interactions that go beyond the job role, which helps team members form more sophisticated relationships. These leaders concern themselves with the quality of interactions between team members, which they expect to be respectful and appropriate, even under duress. They prepare their teams for the inevitable presence of conflict and coach individuals through it when it arises. Perhaps most importantly, successful leaders recognize and remove toxic personnel who disrupt or damage the team's ability to function at a high level.

RELATIONSHIPS BETWEEN TEAMMATES ARE IMPORTANT

The reality of going to work every day means that employees spend as much, if not more, time with co-workers than with family. Human beings are social creatures, so it makes sense that over time sophisticated relationships develop. A case can be made, though, that physicians and managers who want to maximize the performance of their team should take steps to facilitate and accelerate the development of these more sophisticated relationships.

When members of a team form meaningful relationships with one another there is a positive impact on engagement and performance. Beyond the quantifiable attributes of a job (salary, benefits, perks, title, etc.) the quality and depth of workplace relationships can have a significant impact on loyalty. Simply put, employees with established, meaningful workplace relationships are less likely to leave.

When individuals form healthy personal relationships with colleagues at work, the impact is quantifiable. Employees who indicate they have a "best friend" at work are more engaged, more productive, have lower turnover, and deliver higher levels of customer service. While only 30% of the workforce say they have a "best friend" at work, this group is seven times as likely to be engaged. *Seven*!

It should be noted that the kind of relationship described as a "best friend" at work may differ from a best friend outside of the workplace. A best friend at work is someone the employee has formed a personal, social relationship with *at work*. It is a person they can turn to during times of stress and challenge. It's someone that can share in accomplishments and celebrations and who cares about the employee as a person. In some cases this relationship may be limited to work time and location.

The presence of collegiality and caring on a team makes that unit more resilient in the face of any number of stressors. Why? Because if I have had the chance to get to know you beyond the role you are in, even slightly, it's more likely that I will respect you, like you, or want to help you. These become powerful attributes in the face of stress, conflict, or difficulty at work. Such relationships make it more likely that the team can adopt a "we're all in this together" approach and avoid a "that's not my job" culture. If your clinic is consistently understaffed, overbooked, or is regularly visited by difficult or combative patients, group cohesion and team spirit are critical to your success.

Building Relationships Between Team Members
In 1965, Bruce Tuckman first published his renowned model of group development. He argued that, through *forming, storming, norming*, and *performing*, teams mature and evolve. At the core of his research, upon which subsequent development models are widely based, is the acknowledgement that team leaders are largely responsible for facilitating team development. Tuckman's model should be required reading for anyone in a leadership role.

Tuckman suggests that teams who experience fun and social interaction develop commitment and unity. Leaders can prompt and even accelerate team development by using targeted, low-risk opportunities for team members to talk and laugh and connect with one another. It's fun...with a purpose. There are a variety of easy ways you can do this for your team.

- **Use teambuilders and icebreakers.** Identify and facilitate short, low-risk activities at team huddles and staff meetings. Showcase the unique personalities, talents, skills, and knowledge of the individuals that make up the team. See the Resource Box in this chapter for some ideas you can use.

- **Celebrate birthdays, babies, and brides**. Set-up a birthday committee on your team or designate one day a month to celebrate all the birthdays in the office or on the unit. Invite people to bring in their favorite birthday treat or have the committee bring them in based on requests from team members. Wedding showers or baby showers (including for grooms and new dads) on site invite colleagues to celebrate happy life events. Pulling people together in this way, even for just a few minutes, fosters connections and caring.

- **Plan a potluck.** Pick a day, once each quarter, and hold a potluck staff lunch. Invite team members to sign up in advance to bring a favorite dish or show off a favorite recipe. Use these gatherings to celebrate real accomplishments or oddball occasions (The 4th Annual Arbor Day Potluck!)

- **Designate a team bulletin board.** Identify space in a visible, backstage area where staff can post notes, personal items, holiday cards, or vacation pictures. Change it up from time to time and make it fun. Example: Ask everyone to bring in a baby picture and hold a "guess the tyke" contest.

- **Form pods**. Research suggests there is great benefit to working in smaller, tight knit work groups. A team size of between 5 and 9 people appears to be the "sweet spot" where group size contributes notably to engagement levels. Provide employees the chance to work in sub-teams or on project committees. Give them input in choosing who they work with to further boost engagement.

Physicians and managers have a responsibility to create an environment employees want to work in. When team members view each other only through the lens of "work," meaningful relationships are less likely to develop. Create regular opportunities for team members to interact and even socialize. Doing so is an investment in team resiliency and collaboration, and increases the likelihood that your team will smile more, disagree less, and stay longer.

Teambuilding Activities for Meetings or Huddles

These activities are meant to be simple, flexible, and effective. The best team building exercises enhance group cohesion through interaction but also help promote greater work performance. Be sure to utilize the debrief (where provided) to maximize the effectiveness of these exercises.

Back-to-Back Drawing

Divide people into pairs and have each pair sit on the floor back to back. Give one person a picture and give their partner a pencil and paper. The person holding the picture will verbally instruct his or her partner to draw the image without telling them what the image actually is. Once a pre-determined time limit (3-5 minutes works) expires, invite the partners to compare the new drawing with the original picture. This exercise helps foster a sense of interdependence between people, examine and improve communication and interpretative skills, and understand the value of trust in a situation where each person lacks all the necessary tools. DEBRIEF: Afterwards, ask the group to share their thoughts on what could be learned from this activity. Identify important lessons learned or new behaviors to adopt (ex. what we say and what others hear aren't always the same, at times we must be thoughtful about our communication in order to be effective, etc.).

Question Jar
Print 20-30 questions on index cards or strips of paper and store them in a large jar that travels to each team meeting. At the start or end of each meeting draw one question from the jar that each team member quickly answers. Questions might include things like: *Tell us what you were like in high school. What's the best vacation you've ever had? Tell us about your hometown. What one product would you refuse to endorse?*

Balloon Bounce
Place the team in a circle where everyone is standing. Introduce one inflated balloon into the circle and explain that they are required to keep the balloon afloat. It cannot hit the floor. If it does, a member of the group is kicked out of the circle. After a few moments, add another balloon, and then another, and so on. Feel free to ask members of the group to answer questions, stand on one leg, tell a joke, count to ten, etc. I've seen this exercise done with groups as small as five and in a ballroom with over 200 people. Just try participating in this activity without laughing. It's almost impossible. DEBRIEF: Afterwards, ask the group to share their thoughts on what could be learned from this activity. Identify important lessons learned or new behaviors to adopt (ex. we can "juggle" more as a team than as individuals, we rely on each other to keep everyone engaged, etc.)

CONFLICT IS NORMAL AND EXPECTED

A few years ago, I was asked to design and implement a series of retreats for a large anesthesiology department of a multi-site academic medical center. The problem? The working relationships between physicians and CRNAs were damaged. Politics, a lack of trust, and a history of discord created an inability to have needed discussions on key issues, including process, scope-of-practice, and the changing landscape of care delivery. In short, there was an obvious need for these colleagues to talk to each other about how they talk to each other.

Over a period of several weeks, a series of half-day retreats were held, bringing together a balanced mix of physicians and CRNAs. A keynote address on dignity and respect served as a springboard to small group breakouts. Facilitated by practitioners, the breakouts compelled participants to explore the nature and quality of team interactions. By the end of these events, participants had spent several hours discussing the atmosphere of the department and the need to collaborate more respectfully.

The results were instantaneous.

For the first time in years, colleagues listened to one another. They acknowledged the unique challenges facing each position. They took ownership of the roles they played in perpetuating a damaged work environment. Post-event surveys clearly showed that attendees valued the chance to discuss concerns and hear varied professional perspectives. Multiple attendees acknowledged "aha" moments and a deeper understanding of their colleagues' points of view. In a few short hours, participants acknowledged specific behaviors they planned to adopt in the interest of improving the culture and performance of the department. In the months following these retreats, physicians and CRNAs cited this dialogue as having had a significant impact on the culture and atmosphere of the department.

As is often the case, providing a structure and forum for colleagues to discuss how they communicate with each other was a critical step to reducing destructive conflict in the workplace.

Team conflict at work is inevitable. The close proximity of employees and the demands of the environment mean that conflict is almost guaranteed. No workplace, no industry, and no team are immune. So before you read any further, take a moment to accept that. It's inevitable. Conflict will always be there and no leader, no matter how gifted, can make it go away entirely. Indeed, helping your team expect and navigate conflict is part of what you signed up for as a leader.

In healthcare, it's not enough to only be concerned with the quality of interactions team members have with patients and families. The quality of the interactions they have with one another has a profound impact on the culture and engagement level of your workforce. Causes of conflict vary and may be hard to identify, but stress can exacerbate it. Perhaps the clinic is regularly understaffed or overbooked. Perhaps the team deals frequently with combative patients or drug-seeking behavior. Regardless of cause, when team members are pushed to their limit on a daily basis they, as a TV show famously said, "stop being polite, and start getting real." Stress, fatigue, and pressure remove our filters. And when infighting, negative attitudes, cliques, backbiting, gossip, and angst are present, team performance and patient care suffers. For these reasons, physicians and managers must take proactive and real-time steps to reduce and address conflict in the healthcare workplace.

Teach Them How To Handle Conflict When It Arises
It is up to leaders to communicate a framework for resolving conflict. This means that teams have a clear understanding of how conflict should be managed and how to work through disagreements professionally.

Examine your expectations for how you want the team to behave in the face of disagreement. How do you expect them to handle conflict? Should they communicate with one another before bringing issues to you? What ground rules are necessary and expected for any interaction? It can be helpful for you to express standards of conduct around conflict and the answers to these questions can help you get started.

Once you have a clearer picture of how you expect personnel to handle conflict, invite their input into the discussion. Gather your team and articulate that conflict is inevitable, shouldn't be ignored, at times can be healthy, and should be addressed in a professional way with an emphasis on courtesy and respect. This dynamic is critical. Strong leaders expect that co-workers' interactions are respectful and appropriate at all times. In fact, they insist on it.

Once you've communicated your foundational expectations explore team member expectations. Develop a staff agreement that outlines guidelines for how co-workers will communicate, interact, and respond when conflict arises. Work toward specific ground rules, agreed upon by everyone, that may include:

- Don't respond angrily; wait until tempers cool before talking or emailing.

- Approach each other directly first before involving others.

- Don't gossip.

- Approach conflict resolution with a common goal in mind: helping patients and maintaining a healthy team atmosphere.

- No yelling or swearing.

- Always treat each other with courtesy and respect.

Compile the content into a document that is posted or shared. Treat the content as a living document and revisit it anytime a new leader assumes responsibility for a team, when new members join a team, or when specific issues of conflict have arisen that prove difficult to discuss or overcome. Expressly state that you will get involved if necessary, but that it's rarely an appropriate first step. Encourage team members to communicate with one another directly when conflict arises.

To get your hands on a step-by-step guide for facilitating a staff agreement, download the Resource Kit at CureForTheCommonLeader.com.

Get Involved When It Is Necessary
On occasions when employees cannot solve their own issues, you may have to get involved. The leader's role can be multifaceted. You may offer to help a single employee prepare for a conversation with a colleague. Offer to give them feedback on their approach or role-play if necessary. Encourage them to manage their emotions and be respectful while also empathizing with the other person. Be sure to follow up a day or two later. This demonstrates your commitment to their success…and makes sure they didn't get cold feet.

In some cases, you may have to meet with all parties involved. If a sit-down meeting becomes necessary or a conflict explodes quickly, the following steps can help you work toward resolution:

1. Remove the employees from the situation. If the conflict is public, send them each to a different private area. Keep the employees separated to quickly diffuse the argument.

2. Give those involved some time to compose themselves then provide each party a chance to explain the problem to you. Sometimes tension can be relieved by just letting each employee air out his complaints. Avoid interrupting, and be sympathetic to the concerns voiced.

3. As appropriate, ask probing, open-ended questions to get to the root cause of the problem. Consider asking: A) How have you attempted to resolve this? B) Why do you think

this is happening? C) What is he/she going to tell me about this conflict that we haven't talked about?

4. After each employee talks to you independently, bring all involved parties together to discuss the situation.

5. Have the involved parties talk to each other, not to you. Set ground rules and encourage them to make "I" statements. For instance, "I understand you are upset, but when these things occur I feel..."

6. Explore root causes of the problem through dialogue. Help those involved better understand when and why the conflict occurs. Identify factors that may be exacerbating the conflict. Be brave enough to explore how leadership may contribute to the conflict as well.

7. Decide on how the situation can be resolved. Attempt to identify a compromise or environmental change to address the problem. Ask: "Where do we go from here?" or "What one action can we agree to take to move forward?"

8. Host a follow-up conversation as needed.

9. If a suitable compromise cannot be found you may need to impose expectations for how interactions should take place going forward.

Conflict is not always bad. Conflict is often an opportunity to enhance communication and produce change that many are collectively invested in. While a lot of advice is offered in this chapter, I should state explicitly that there is no right, clear, or perfect way to handle conflict when it occurs, or to change a team culture. Nobody has THE answer when it comes to the complex sum of emotion, behavior, and perception that typically fuels conflict. But if you take proactive steps to set expectations before conflict arises, then, when it inevitably does, guide team members through an even-keeled, open dialogue heavy on courtesy and respect, you will be successful more often than not.

TOXIC FORCES MUST BE REMOVED

In my career I've worked with a great many practices and groups burdened with challenging interpersonal issues. I have been asked to help with teams that yell and scream at each other, that aren't on speaking terms, and teams where personnel wouldn't stay for more than a short period of time because the environment was so harsh. When approached to assist with these and other staff conflict issues, I start with a single question:

"Is there one person on your team that, if they were to leave, your problems would largely go away, too?"

At least half the time the answer is "Yes."

"Then you don't have a problem that training will solve," I say. "You have a performance management problem that you need to address with the individual."

When bad behavior is not addressed it can be cancerous to a team. If a toxic personality is present, leadership must engage in focused, specific, behavioral conversations about what that person needs to do differently. If that has occurred and no improvement follows, leadership must take appropriate steps, in collaboration with a Human Resources professional, to remove that employee. Period. Unfortunately, though, many teams turn this kind of black and white issue into a grey one.

Over and over again, I hear this story: "We have one nurse who is a bit rough around the edges. She is pushy and negative and snaps at people sometimes. Many of the staff walk on eggshells around her. But she does her job really well and is a great nurse…"

No, she is not a "great nurse."

A "great nurse" wouldn't exhibit such behavior. A "great nurse" is the total package- technically skilled and collegial. Why so many seem willing to tolerate questionable interpersonal behavior from those who are technically sound is beyond me. In this example, if the performance was reversed - the nurse was approachable and collaborative but was technically deficient - most organizations would address that without hesitation. Why are so many willing to tolerate poor interpersonal conduct, when interpersonal conduct so directly impacts every facet of a patient care environment?

When leaders fail to address inappropriate, disrespectful, or negative employee behavior, the team suffers. This is where teams need leaders to take clear, decisive action. When presented with an employee whose style or approach is cancerous to the team, clearly inform the employee that their behavior is not meeting expectations. If the negative behavior continues, then that person should not be allowed to continue as a member of the team.

Eighteen percent of the workforce is Actively Disengaged. These employees make more errors, restrict productivity, and monopolize a leader's time. They have more time and attendance issues, damage your reputation, and suck the life out of your team. They undermine all that you and others are trying to accomplish. They stand in the way of achieving the level of service delivery and team performance that you aspire to every day. Actively Disengaged employees are weeds in a garden. No matter how many beautiful flowers are present or how much fertilizer you use, the weed will always be a weed, and it will mar your landscape until it is removed.

Removing the Actively Disengaged

If an Actively Disengaged employee is present on your team, you must embark on a journey to improve their performance or remove them from the team. There are no other options.

Start with a feedback conversation. Identify the specific behaviors the employee is using that need to stop. Identify the new behaviors the employee must display going forward. Be clear. Your conversation should include specific examples of problematic behavior and expected improvements. Document the conversation, share a summary with the employee, and plan to follow up in a relatively short period of time. Many human resources professionals can help you install a formal performance improvement plan that holds the staff member accountable to specific changes across an agreed upon time frame. (For more on giving performance feedback, see Chapter 8).

Invite the employee's input on their goals and interests in an effort to promote engagement. Admittedly, there is a limit to the amount of change or accommodation you can make to spark improved performance.

Explore with the employee the aspects of their work they find fulfilling and energizing. Identify the unique strengths and talents they possess and examine whether it is possible to position them to use them more frequently in their role. Identify those forces at work that seemingly contribute to the disengagement the employee exhibits. A handful of conversations will likely clarify for you, as the leader, whether rehabilitation (for lack of a better word) is a possibility.

These steps to convert the employee's negative performance are required. They reflect the due diligence, morally and legally, that leaders must do to exhaust all options before separating an employee from a position. For many Actively Disengaged employees, however, this separation is inevitable and necessary. My experience has been that past performance is the best predictor of future performance. There are simply some people who are predisposed to toxic workplace behavior. If no possibility of change is evident or no improvement occurs, these employees must be removed without hesitation, if for no other reason than to demonstrate to the larger team that certain expectations related to interpersonal communication, collaboration, and outlook are highly valued and must be met.

Employees learn and replicate what they experience. When poisonous personalities are allowed to remain, their behavior becomes a part of "how we do things around here." In the end their presence sabotages the performance of others, the atmosphere of the work environment, and the quality of care delivered to patients.

In other words: pull the weeds.

WHAT PHYSICIANS AND MANAGERS MUST DO TO FOSTER GROUP COHESION AND TEAM SPIRIT

Action Items Summary:
- Provide employees with opportunities to develop sophisticated relationships with co-workers.

- Use teambuilders and icebreakers to prompt low-risk social interaction between teammates.

- Celebrate birthdays, babies, and weddings to foster connections and caring.

- Hold an occasional staff lunch or potluck. Involve staff in planning and executing.

- Find ways to give employees a chance to work in small teams or "pods."

- Install a framework for resolving conflict. Review your expectations and invite the team to outline guidelines for how to handle conflict when it occurs.

- Help prepare employees for difficult conversations with peers.

- Mediate conflict that employees are unable to resolve individually.

- Hold team members accountable for the quality of interactions they have with one another. Insist on the constant presence of courtesy and respect.

- Address employees whose interpersonal conduct is inappropriate or damages the team. Communicate a clear performance improvement plan that outlines expected behavior.

- If disruptive, toxic, or negative employees fail to improve, remove them from the team as quickly as possible.

Chapter 6

You Must Connect Each Employee To A Powerful Purpose

Dr. Enheim assembled his team in the small conference room at the back of the practice. An oncology clinic with a women's health focus, his team consisted of front-desk personnel, medical assistants, nurses, two Physician Assistants, a surgery scheduler and a practice manager. After thanking everyone for making time after another busy day, he turned to the person sitting directly to his left and asked a question.

"Sue…what is your job?"

Looking confused, Sue answered, "I'm a Medical Assistant."

"That's your title," Dr. Enheim replied. "What's your *job*?" he asked. "What do you *do*?

"Um…well…I room patients. I take their vitals. I handle labs…"

Dr. Enheim moved to the next employee at the table, a Physician Assistant. "What's your job, Dana?" he asked.

"I'm a PA," Dana replied. "I see patients, conduct exams, prescribe medication, and work with you and our other physicians to administer a care plan."

Around the table Dr. Enheim went. After everyone in the room finished answering his "What's your job?" question, he folded his arms.

"I owe you an apology," he said. "I have been remiss in my duties as a leader in this practice. I haven't taken the necessary steps to help you understand what your job really is."

Confused faces stared back at him.

He pressed on. "Because any time anybody ever asks you the question 'What's your job?' there is only one answer. It's the same for each and every one of us. And I hope that, from this point forward and for as long as you work here, you will answer that question with only three words."

He turned and wrote on the dry erase board at the front of the room. When he stepped away, his team stared at the short phrase.

"I cure cancer."

THE POWER OF PURPOSE

When I met with Dr. Enheim and his practice manager, they detailed several challenges facing their team. They described a kind of class system among the staff. The front-desk workers complained that the MAs and nurses talked down to them. The MAs and nurses complained that the PAs talked down to *them*. Most everyone in the office had some complaint or another about a different staff member who never did what they were supposed to. "That's not my job" was a refrain heard frequently around the clinic. As our conversation progressed, we all agreed there was a lack of respect for the differing roles each employee played in delivering services, caring for patients, and supporting each other.

I designed the exercise above, with Dr. Enheim going around the room and asking each employee to answer the question, "What's your job?" to help the team begin a conversation about the ways they were dependent on one another. Part reflection activity and part theatre, Dr. Enheim's goal was to establish a powerful purpose central to everyone's work.

"I cure cancer" is an incredibly powerful purpose.

"This is what we do here. Each of us," he told his team that day. "Sue, your job is to cure cancer. You do it by rooming patients, taking their vitals, handling labs, etc. Dana, you do it by seeing patients and conducting exams and executing care plans. But you can't do it without her," he said as he pointed toward Sue. "And you can't do it without her," he said, pointing back to Dana. And around the table he went once again, highlighting the interdependence necessary to do what everyone was there to do: cure cancer.

In the weeks and months following, I helped Dr. Enheim and his practice manager identify ways to build upon the powerful conversation that took place that day. Over time the interactions between team members improved. Things didn't change overnight. But the leadership team in that clinic landed upon a potent concept that resonated with everyone and that they kept as the central focus of all conversations.

As noted in the first chapter, many, many organizations are studying workplace engagement and the factors that contribute to its presence. Were you to comb through the piles of research on the subject or examine the hundreds of engagement models marketed by experts around the world, you would come to the realization that at the core of engagement is purpose.

Employees have to believe their work matters. That they contribute to something meaningful. Where leaders rally team members to a cause greater than self, engagement levels are consistently high. It is not overly simplistic to suggest that leadership effectiveness comes predominantly from the ability to articulate a clear, powerful reason employees should care and try. Show me a successful leader, at any level, and I will show you someone who gives voice to purpose and makes an effort to keep it in the spotlight day in and day out.

Purpose is central to engagement. That's why this chapter may be the most important one in this book.

Behaviors are informed by emotions. To inspire employees to work hard, get along, and wow patients, leaders have to create line of sight between the tasks and responsibilities of employees' jobs and a powerful purpose that stirs the emotions. When this purpose is absent, employees simply execute tasks. They go through the motions. Research supports the need for leaders to articulate a big picture meaning for employees and tie it to the work they do. In a 2012 survey of multiple industries, only 41% of employees felt they knew what their company stands for and what makes its brand different from its competitors'.

Identifying Your Purpose

To get started, answer this question: What is the powerful purpose at the core of everything your site does? For many in healthcare the first answer is, "We help sick people get better." While this is true, it's not clear or expressive enough. Leaders must dig deeper to come up with language that touches those who do the work. I spend extensive time on this in workshops and at retreats, pushing participants until they land upon dramatic language for their individual sites. I've watched the leadership team of a fertility clinic beam with pride as they finally articulated their powerful purpose: "We make dreams come true." I've sat with nurse managers who became emotional when talking about the freedom and dignity they give back to the patients in their urogynecology clinic. That became the core purpose they championed: "We give these women their freedom and dignity back." After discussing all the ways colds, injuries, and a lack of wellness disrupts the daily lives of most who experience them, I watched the staff of a small primary care clinic thrill at acknowledging their powerful purpose: "We get lives back on track."

As an individual, a leadership team, or as a staff, begin a conversation about your team's powerful purpose. As you come up with answers keep asking the question "Why is that important?" Drill down to a sentiment or mantra that stops you in your tracks. Don't be afraid to reach for lofty language. It's almost impossible to not experience feelings of pride and purpose when you're given permission to tell the world: "I cure cancer." Give everyone who works for you a purpose that is impossible to dismiss. You will know when you've landed on the right language for your site. You will probably get goose bumps.

Line of Sight

Once you have settled on language that articulates your purpose you must find ways to connect that purpose to the day-to-day work of your employees. There are several ways leaders do this.

- **Say it constantly**. Give voice to your purpose over and over again. Work it into meetings, team huddles, and emails. Get to the point where the staff knows it's coming before you say it. That's not a bad thing.

- **Answer "why" questions with purpose, not performance goals**. When explaining the reasons for taking (or not taking) an action, complying with a policy, or initiating a change, tie the reasons for doing so to your purpose. Example: employees must complete annual mandatory training to stay informed and continue providing the best care possible. Not because "it's required."

- **Highlight during onboarding.** Make new team members aware of your purpose right away. It is one of the most important things they learn early on. Show them evidence of the impact they can have in their role.

- **Move from task orientation to purpose orientation**. Connect even basic job duties to your powerful purpose. Leaders do this by assigning responsibilities, not tasks. For example, don't assign someone to stuff envelopes. Instead, give them the responsibility for notifying your patients about your location change via mail. Grant authority to increase ownership and accountability.

- **Highlight one-on-one**. Point out to individual employees how their efforts manifested your powerful purpose. Leave notes, pull people aside, and mention it in one-on-one meetings. Be specific. Do this often.

- **Include in feedback conversations**. When addressing performance issues explain how the undesired or incorrect behavior demonstrated by the employee fails to fulfill your purpose.

- **Give physical reminders**. Put your purpose on a mug. Post it on your refrigerator, at the bottom of staff meeting agendas, or in cards and notes. If appropriate for patients to see, pass out buttons or stickers to add to ID badges.

- **Use activities and exercises to illustrate and reinforce**. For a free copy of a 20-minute "patient-centered care" staff development activity, get the free *Cure for the Common Leader* Resource Kit at CureForTheCommonLeader.com.

Become a Storyteller

The most effective way leaders cultivate purpose among employees is by constantly sharing examples of the ways in which their work makes a difference. Put another way: great leaders are great story-tellers.

This is perhaps best illustrated by the challenging confrontation Emily Wilson had with a patient's spouse in the waiting room of her hospital-based clinic. The patient, a 68-year-old woman with head and neck cancer, arrived for her appointment with her husband in tow. When the doctor met with the patient he quickly realized she had been scheduled into an appointment at the wrong location. In tandem with the front-desk staff, he returned her co-pay and made arrangements for the patient to be seen at the proper location, with the appropriate specialist, across town later that day. When a staff member explained the mix up to the patient, her husband lost his cool. In the waiting room, for all to see, he began yelling obscenities at the staff and demanded to see the manager. When Emily appeared, the husband got right in her face. Emily apologized repeatedly and invited both parties back to her office, but the husband refused. He explicitly stated that he wanted to make a scene. The staff present and others in the waiting room were subjected to an unsettling and tense interaction. Emily remained calm throughout, never raising her voice or becoming defensive. After several minutes the husband calmed down and Emily walked them through the details of how to get where they needed to go.

I'll let Emily tell you what happened next.

"My staff were shaken. They watched the whole thing unfold. He really came at me and they were worried about me. Once the couple left, I pulled my team together to debrief what had happened. When they asked me how I stayed so calm, I told them, 'His wife has cancer. He's scared to death. His complaint has nothing to do with having to drive to another appointment. His complaint truly is that his wife has cancer. His way of dealing with it in that moment was to yell at people. Because he can't yell at cancer. So I let him yell.'"

With a few sentences, Emily got her team to trade their defensiveness for empathy. In those few sentences, she created line of sight between the difficult situation her team faced and a powerful purpose that accessed their compassion. Cultivating purpose for your team means arming them with empathy.

There are four kinds of stories leaders can tell to give employees perspective and trigger compassion, empathy, and resilience.

- **Impact on patients**. Describe how the actions or efforts of the employee have a positive effect on patients as individuals or as a group. Example: "We have to be fully staffed 30 minutes before the first appointment in case there's an emergent situation. Like what happened to Mrs. Jones last week."

- **Impact on teammates**. Point out how the employee's work positively impacted other members of the team. Example: "Because you took on these additional duties, the entire nursing staff got out on time. Had you not helped, they would all have had to stay late."

- **Important cog in the machine**. It's important to remind employees from time to time that their work has a far-reaching ripple effect. Example: "Because you took care of Dr. Wilson's CME paperwork, he was able to see three more patients today, all of whom certainly appreciated not having to wait another day for an appointment."

- **Hypothetical loved one**. Leaders can reinforce the right way of doing things by simply asking, "If it was your mother/daughter/grandfather, how would you want them to be treated?"

These kinds of stories should be woven into your interactions with team members. They should also be used when answering "why" questions. In all your interactions, support team members actions and effort with reasons that access their empathy. Learn to do this consistently, and your team members will be more inspired to produce effort after talking with you.

While it's important to identify a powerful purpose for employees, and it's equally important to spell out the ways their work helps others, employees must also believe their work is valued by leaders and teammates. This is why physicians and managers must also provide employee recognition on a continual basis.

YOU BETTER RECOGNIZE

What do you think of when you hear the term "employee recognition?" I asked this question to a group of managers and physicians during an extended leadership training course. As part of a word-association exercise, they made this list:

- *Awards*

- *Perks*

- *Prizes*

- *Gifts*

- *Reward*

- *Nominate*

- *Performance Bonus*

- *Card*

- *Advancement*

- *Positive Feedback*

- *Program*

- *Thank you*

- *Certificate*

- *Gift cards*

- *Appreciation*

- *Team lunch*

Let's face it…that's a lousy list.

Contrary to what that list suggests, employee recognition has very little to do with awards, gifts, and other physical manifestations of appreciation. Employee recognition is not about what the employee receives. It's about the *feelings* they experience.

Acknowledging contributions, effort, talents, or skills in such a way that the employee experiences feelings of appreciation is central to engagement. When this intentional communication of the ways employees achieve, matter, help, and contribute to a greater purpose is continuously present, productivity, performance, resiliency, and retention are high. Dissatisfaction, disengagement, and turnover are low.

That's why the list above is a lousy list. The items listed focus on the delivery system used for recognition, not the sentiment - the expression of gratitude and appreciation and the subsequent feelings it produces for the employee. Formal recognition programs often suffer from this disconnect. That's not to say formal programs and external rewards aren't effective. They can be, as long as the emphasis remains on the acknowledgment of the specific ways the employee makes a difference. Recognition that leads to engagement occurs not through the occasional distribution of gifts or perks, but by taking time and using words to notice, acknowledge, and praise.

Frequent, Simple, and Specific

To impact engagement, recognition efforts that intentionally highlight the value and contribution of team members must be continuous. Employees must regularly see and hear the ways they make a difference to those around them. This kind of ongoing recognition is a core strategy for creating line of sight between employees and a purpose greater than themselves. Effective employee recognition then doesn't occur as singular, grand gestures, but as continuous, habitual conversations that take place frequently. How frequently, you ask? Science has an answer.

Research in workplace positivity by psychologist Dr. Marcia Losada found that the most effective teams have more positive interactions. There is even a number that corresponds to the minimum amount of positive to negative feedback necessary to encourage successful functioning: three positive remarks for every negative one. Keep this 3-to-1 ratio in mind when balancing recognition and constructive feedback. Strive to direct positive comments to employees at least three times as often as you direct corrective or procedural feedback.

This is where physicians and managers are critical to success. You are the only people in the work-life of the employee with both the power and opportunity to recognize employees (that is, to celebrate their value) on a regular basis. Think about it:

- Who sees employee behavior, performance, and contributions most frequently?

- Who is the organizational "authority-figure" to the employee?

- Who conducts the formal evaluation of employee performance?

- Who is charged with leading the team?

- Who sets the tone of the work environment? The culture? The atmosphere?

- Who connects employees to upper management and executives?

The role you play in using recognition as a strategy for cultivating purpose cannot be overstated. Frequent and targeted recognition is a key leadership strategy that must be embraced by managers and physicians at all levels to actively engage the workforce. You must do it, because no one else *can*.

Recognition efforts don't have to be grand gestures and they don't have to take a lot of time. Remember, the goal is to present evidence of impact and stir feelings of worth and appreciation within the employee. Set aside 15 to 30 minutes a week to plan and/or execute recognition and it will begin to become a habit. Not sure what to do or how to do it? Look for the Resource Box in this chapter for 17 ways to recognize that take less than 15 minutes a day.

Note also that you do not need a spectacular accomplishment or a formal occasion to engage in recognition. Celebrating small victories, accomplishments, or contributions can have a huge impact on the morale of individuals and teams. Point out when something has been done well. Say, "Thank you." Do it often...and include everyone.

Celebrate and Involve Everyone

Imagine you came to one of my management training programs and, prior to its start, I offered you a choice of the following door prizes: a water bottle, a rubber band, or an iPad. Without hesitation, most would choose the iPad, right? Clearly it's the most valuable item of the three. It's flashy, slick, and contemporary. It is the superstar of the group. The iPad stands out in stark contrast to the other two items, which aren't even in the same league.

This happens in teams as well. It is easy to recognize the superstars. They stand out. They bring something obvious to the group and as a leader, you don't have to work hard to recognize them. But not everyone is a superstar.

Had you taken a few moments to examine the water bottle, you would have found a sturdy, reliable device. It never leaks, it's portable, consistent, and is always there when you need it. And the rubber band? Invaluable. It is strong, flexible, and can handle quite a lot of stress.

And neither will *ever* be an iPad.

Recognition is about celebrating the unique talents and contributions of every member of a team. It's easy to lose sight of these gifts if employees work daily in the shadow of a high performer, but most employees bring something to the table. Take time to figure out what that is and celebrate it. Whether it's administrative responsibilities, interpersonal interactions with clients, or how they relate to their co-workers, celebrate everyone, and help them see how their "routine" contributions produce powerful results.

Recognition from leaders isn't the only way to stir feelings of appreciation and impact. Peer recognition also impacts an employee's sense of purpose. When individual contributors get praise from peers, they believe they are needed. They believe they contribute.

Invite your team to identify ways to acknowledge one another. When someone mentions to you that they benefited from the effort or talent of another on the team, strongly encourage that person to write a note, say thank you, or acknowledge the helper at an upcoming meeting. In some settings, peer-to-peer recognition ends up being the most powerful form of recognition. That's why several of the 17 ideas in this chapter's Resource Box involve peers.

17 SIMPLE WAYS TO RECOGNIZE EMPLOYEES THAT COMMUNICATE VALUE AND IMPACT

1. A handwritten card

2. Thank you emails

3. Leave a post-it note

4. When working long or extra hours, send a thank you note home to the family

5. Highlight in performance evaluation

6. Invite to train others

7. Compose a letter for employment file

8. Gift idea: Book with an inscribed note

9. Highlight specific employee performance to senior executives

10. Acknowledge performance in a newsletter, staff email update, announcements, etc.

11. Provide customers opportunities to share their positive experiences and display accordingly

12. Invite employee to present at a meeting

13. Invite employee to present to senior executives

14. Invite a senior executive to a staff meeting to highlight employee accomplishments

15. Have staff share "kudos" at meetings, publicly acknowledging help they received from teammates

16. Give the team Lifesavers candies to hand out to one another to acknowledge each other

17. Create an office trophy or mascot that can be awarded weekly or monthly

Recognition reinforces the kind of performance and behaviors you want consistently out of your employees. High job performance is a learned behavior. Emotional rewards, in the form of recognition and validation, provide reinforcement to that ongoing learning. So too does exposure to a powerful purpose and evidence of contribution to that purpose.

WHAT PHYSICIANS AND MANAGERS MUST DO TO CONNECT EMPLOYEES TO PURPOSE

Action Items Summary:

- Work with your leadership team or staff as a whole to identify a powerful purpose that is at the core of everything your site does.

- Use clear, expressive language that stirs the emotions.

- Give voice to your powerful purpose over and over again.

- Include your purpose in team meetings, one-on-one conversations, new hire training, and feedback dialogue.

- Delegate responsibilities, not just tasks, to increase ownership and accountability.

- Give out or post physical reminders of your purpose to remind and reinforce.

- Share stories that highlight how employees' work contributes to a larger purpose.

- Engage in ongoing recognition that specifically communicates value and impact to evoke feelings of worth and appreciation.

- Strive for a 3-to-1 ratio of positive feedback and constructive criticism.

- Set aside 15 to 30 minutes a week to plan and execute recognition efforts.

- Recognize the contributions of everyone, not just your superstars.

Chapter 7
You Must Hire And Onboard Intentionally

Ever notice that most new hires display many of the characteristics of Engaged employees? They arrive eager to learn and hungry to make a difference. They put forth effort and are willing to do what it takes. Depending on their level of social comfort, many actively start working to get to know teammates and build relationships. This isn't just perception. Research suggests that workers are typically more engaged in their first 3-6 months on the job than at any other stage in their employment.

So what happens?

Why do the naturally occurring engagement levels that come with being new start to wane? What causes Engaged workers to evolve into Not Engaged or Actively Disengaged workers? Certainly the absence of many of the conditions outlined in this book cause employees to devolve in this way. Disengagement, however, is accelerated if an effective, thoughtful hiring and onboarding process does not occur.

Employees who remain engaged over the long term experience several key happenings when they interview, accept a job, and arrive at their new workplace. When these things transpire, it increases the likelihood of sustained engagement for that employee. The absence of these events can quickly turn what would otherwise be a valuable contributor into a disaffected short-timer.

In other words, the courtship and the honeymoon make the marriage.

How you identify and intake new personnel play a significant role in facilitating and sustaining engagement. This chapter will help you examine your current processes and identify the things you must do, right out of the gate, to set people up for success.

HIRING

Hooray! You finally received approval to add another position to your team. Perhaps your site is expanding or a hiring freeze has been lifted. Maybe you are simply replacing an employee who left for greener pastures.

The harried demands of healthcare often push leaders into approaching the hiring process with one goal in mind: get a new person as fast as possible. This priority on speed isn't necessarily bad, but too often it leads to oversights in other critical areas. Are they a good fit for the rest of the team? For the patient population? For the responsibilities of the position? For the leadership style of the physicians and managers?

Taking even a small amount of time to thoughtfully approach the hiring process increases the chances that you will ultimately hire someone with the right mix of talent, knowledge, skill, and personality. You will also need to bring your patience, because finding the right person almost never happens as quickly as you hope.

Ask the Right Questions
Job interviews provide employers and potential employees the opportunity to evaluate each other. The employer is evaluating the candidate both in terms of technical expertise and personality, while the employee is exploring the dynamics of the work environment and whether the position meets their wants and needs. The questions you ask a potential employee go a long way towards deter-

mining whether or not you will learn what you need to learn about that candidate. This is why behavioral-based interview questions are best.

For decades, job interviews consisted of questions that led to hypothetical, idealized responses ("How would you handle..."). Candidates told employers what they wanted to hear in the hopes of getting the job. Upon hiring, they may or may not possess the requisite skills and experience to succeed in the role. It wasn't until more recently that employers recognized the need to draw out actual experiences of candidates to better evaluate their suitability for a position. Enter behavioral-based interviewing.

Behavioral-based interview questions ask interviewees to recall actual situations and describe their choices and behaviors. The person asking the question typically starts out with, *"Tell me about a time when..."* and then describes a challenge or problem the candidate might face in their new role. For example: *"Tell me about a time when you had to juggle many competing responsibilities at once."*

This approach is based on the belief that past performance is the best predictor of future behavior. In fact, behavioral interviewing is said to be 55% predictive of future on-the-job behavior, while traditional interviewing is only 10% predictive.

In the ensuing dialogue the interviewer can ask follow-up questions such as, *"What actions did you take?"* and *"What was the outcome?"* to draw out the whole story. In general, behavioral questions allow the interviewer to glean additional information from the actions the candidate describes (there's a certain amount of reading between the lines that occurs when conducting behavioral-based interviews). For example, if a candidate describes how she deescalated an angry patient in the waiting room, one could infer that she was comfortable facing those kinds of interactions. If she instead stated that her first step was to get the manager, one could deduce the candidate is less confident in the face of difficult behavior. As the candidate describes how she went about service recovery, the interviewer might infer that she has received customer service training of some kind, prompting a follow up question regarding her specific training in that area. Behavioral-based interviewing allows you to explore tangible, real-life situations a potential employee has handled, as well as their instincts, demeanor, skills, and personality.

You can easily come up with a list of behavioral-based questions by identifying desired skills and behaviors of the ideal candidate, and then structuring open-ended questions and statements to elicit detailed responses. For example, if your new hire needs to be able to rebuff drug-seeking behavior, you can start out by asking, *"Tell me about a time when you had to tell a customer something they didn't want to hear."*

In addition to exploring skills and behaviors, you must also ascertain *fit*. While "fit" is perhaps one of the vaguest words used in recruitment and selection, successful leaders tune into whether or not the candidate will be a good fit for the team, job role, manager, and organization. During the interview, be sure to ask about career aspirations and what appeals to the candidate about the position and organization. Not sure what to ask? Don't worry. I've got you covered. For a list of 12 questions EVERY candidate for a healthcare job should answer, see the Resource Box in this chapter.

Tell the Unvarnished Truth

Have you ever interviewed for and accepted a job only to arrive and find that it bore no resemblance to the job you were expecting? I bet you felt angry...or duped.

12 Questions Every Candidate
For A Healthcare Job Should Answer

1. What appeals to you about the work you'll be doing in this position?

2. Tell me about a time when you were confronted with a difficult patient or customer. How did you handle it?

3. When were you most satisfied at a job?

4. Tell me about a time when you had to juggle multiple time-sensitive priorities at once. How did you do it?

5. Share a time when you had to follow a policy or process you didn't agree with? What were the results?

6. Tell me about a time when you made a significant mistake at work. How did you handle it?

7. Describe a time when you had to bend the rules to achieve a goal. What was the outcome?

8. Describe the most stressful day at work you've ever had. How did you cope?

9. Tell me about a time when you had to work with a demanding leader or teammate. What was your approach?

10. Why are you looking to leave your current position?

11. If I asked your former colleagues to share a story with us that highlighted your strengths, what story would they tell?

12. What are your long-term career aspirations?

Don't forget to leave time for the candidate to ask questions. In fact, the quality of the questions candidates ask can also tell you a lot about their suitability for the position.

I bet it significantly impacted your engagement in that position.

In the constant quest to staff sites quickly and with the strongest possible performers, it is common for physicians and managers to paint a rosy picture of the job role and work environment. At the very least they shy away from details that might turn off a potential hire. This whitewashing does nothing but set up the new hire to experience a variety of negative emotions upon arrival, especially if they will work in a challenging setting.

What if, instead of glossing over the unappealing stuff, you told the unvarnished truth?

What if, during interviews with candidates, you laid out exactly what was both good and challenging about the role? What would happen if you described that the new hire had to be able to serve multiple demanding physicians who yell a lot? Or that they would rarely get their choice of shift in their first year because of seniority in scheduling? What if you told the candidate, "The phones ring non-stop and the voices on the other end can be nasty. I need someone with a thick skin."

Will the unsanitized truth push some candidates away? Of course. But you don't want those people for employees anyway. They, in all likelihood, would not be the right fit for the job. However, when a candidate hears the truth and accepts the position anyway, they come into the role with their eyes wide open. They know what to expect. You also begin to earn their respect early, because you were unflinchingly honest with them.

I recently led a workshop for physicians and managers on how they can affect culture change on their teams. Near the start of that program I moved participants through an exercise to accurately describe their culture. One woman, an experienced office manager of a small outpatient lab, described her culture thusly:

"We are a team of seven, doing the work of eleven, in a space built for five. We are on top of each other and constantly under siege. Most days are hard, but we try to make it fun for each other and we take pride in handling it all. We're small but mighty."

I loved her answer. I asked her if she would ever use that description when describing the work environment to a candidate for employment. She hesitated, admitting that her reluctance came from knowing it might turn off a good candidate. However it didn't take long for everyone in the room, including the office manager, to realize how powerful her honest description would be in finding the right person to join her team.

So do what your mom always told you to do: Tell the truth.

Get Ready

Once an offer has been accepted by a candidate, there is still important work to do. The steps you take in the time between hiring and arrival determine how smooth and thorough the onboarding process will be for your new employee.

After a candidate has accepted the position, call them to express your excitement that they are joining your team. Reinforce their decision to join your organization. This is especially important if you did not make the job offer to the candidate and haven't spoken with them since the interview. If there is a Human Resources department in your organization that facilitates the hiring steps, make it a point to reach out to the new hire as soon as you become aware they have accepted the position. This is also a chance for you to share anything they need to know in advance of their first day, including shift start and end times, where they should report for work, and dress code. Never assume others have covered this information. Before ending the call, give the new hire a phone number or email address where they can reach you in the event they have questions prior to arrival.

Make a point to announce the new hire to your team. Tell them about their new colleague. Spotlight some of the reasons he or she was selected for the role. Demonstrate enthusiasm for the person joining and you will generate excitement among the team. Remind them that while help is on the way, everyone will need to assist with getting the new hire comfortable and competent in their new job. Encourage the team to be helpful and patient ("Remember everyone, we were all new once.").

At this point, you can ask for volunteers (or assign these duties, but volunteers are always better) to aid in the onboarding of your new hire. Several steps must be taken to ensure a smooth transition for the new employee. Team members can take an active role in preparing for and orienting a new hire in these ways:

- Cleaning and prepping their workspace

- Training the new hire on processes, software, equipment, etc.

- Giving a tour of the site

- Taking the new hire to lunch on the first day

- Allowing the new hire to shadow them during orientation

- Being their designated mentor during the orientation period

Begin assembling a training schedule for the new employee's first one to two weeks. Involve as many team members as possible. This spreads the workload across several individuals and provides the new employee the chance to begin meeting and building relationships with team members. As soon as the new employee is hired, initiate the technical steps necessary to create accounts for email and software programs, as these things often take time. In general, look ahead to everything the employee will need to perform the job and make every effort to have it in place for their first day on the job. Want to make sure you stay on top of everything? Head over to CureForTheCommonLeader.com and download the free Resource Kit, which includes a *Physicians and Managers Checklist for Welcoming New Employees.*

ONBOARDING

"We're all really excited that you're here, Joe. Why don't you go into your office and start going through the files in your desk?"

This was the entirety of my orientation.

Six years into my career, I accepted a position designing and delivering health education training programs as part of the medical center of a major research university. I'll never forget the feelings of confusion and helplessness as I stood up and exited my new boss's office. Go through the files in my desk? And do what with them, exactly?

I spent the following weeks orienting myself to the position. I set up meetings with personnel I thought would be key stakeholders and business partners for me in my role. I initiated weekly meetings with my new boss to ask hundreds of questions, identify her needs and goals for me in the position, and better understand the systems and processes used in the office. The departments and colleagues I partnered with were incredibly helpful. My new boss, the Director of the office where I worked, was not. Much of the time I was given little direction, or told, "We tried that before, it won't work." Eventually I stopped asking, and started doing.

107

Six months later, after years of failing to meet expectations in the role, my boss was terminated from her position.

I was asked to take her place. Six months into my new job, I was running an office with seven employees that served over 30,000 students.

I was 27 years old.

My story is an all too common one. Employee gets hired, arrives at their new job, and gets little training and support transitioning into the position. Admittedly, my story took a very different turn than most. Often, the new hire's feelings of frustration, worthlessness, or anger drive them to leave, or they suffer in silence. For those employees who stay, this can be the origin of disengagement.

Leaders have a responsibility and an obligation to assist new employees with acclimating into their new roles. This is another area of management for which many leaders receive little training. If you have benefited from hands-on supervisors who guided you through a robust orientation and training as part of a new job, you will likely do the same for others. If you were left to fend for yourself, you may leave others to do the same. When the Center for Creative Leadership asked healthcare employees about the capabilities of their leaders, "too narrow a functional orientation" was cited as the biggest area of weakness. Too many supervisors do not know how to onboard effectively, or don't set aside enough time to do so. But the research in this area is clear: the more effort and attention you put forth to train and support a new hire, the more likely it is they will be one of the 30% of employees engaged in their work.

The First Day
I am fortunate to have experienced both ineffective and ideal first days on the job. Four years after accepting the position described earlier, I left the university and accepted a learning and develop-

ment position with a world-renowned academic medical center. My orientation to that position, and the role my new supervisor played, were dramatically different than what I experienced in the previous job. On my first day I received a detailed, two-week training schedule. It was immediately clear that my new boss, and the team she led, had taken great steps to prepare for my arrival. In addition to knowing what was expected, I felt welcomed and valued. This was but one of many things I experienced in my first three months on the job that allowed me to be highly successful in that role.

The first day on the job is your chance to get the employee started off on the right foot. As noted previously, make sure their space is ready for them. It should be clean, stocked with necessary supplies, and include all the equipment and materials they need to do their job. Make sure their computer works and that no defects in the furniture are present. Consider posting a welcome sign celebrating their arrival.

In the early part of the day, arrange for the new hire to receive a tour of the facilities. Identify a team member to walk them around (or do this yourself) and introduce them to colleagues and key contacts. Make sure the providers on site get introduced as well. Unfamiliar faces can be off-putting in the midst of care delivery. If your practice has multiple sites, take the new employee to meet the other teams and see the other facilities.

Once you have completed a general orientation of the work environment, it's time to begin discussing the employee's first few weeks on the job. Set aside one-on-one time with the employee to review this information on the first day. Provide a printed copy of their job description and go through it in detail. Review the training schedule you've created and outline what they will learn in the days and weeks ahead. Take time to outline what you expect them to accomplish and in what time frame. Set two or three specific learning goals for their first few weeks. This helps the new employee understand what your priorities are, and positions them to adopt the same priorities.

During this first conversation, take time to describe the powerful purpose they fill in their job. As you've read already, creating line of sight between an employee's job and a powerful purpose is critical to fostering motivation and engagement. Describe your patient population. Share stories of the ways your team makes a difference in the lives of others. Foreshadow the impact they will have. Giving voice to their purpose early, and reinforcing it during their first months on the job, will help them weather the stress of being new.

Since, in addition to becoming technically proficient in the job, you want the new hire to acclimate to the team, identify ways for them to begin interacting with others right away. I always like to take new hires out to lunch on the first day. Make some others on the team available to participate as well. Be friendly and social and talk about anything BUT the job. Get to know the person joining the group and give them a chance to get to know others. Be careful not to turn that lunch into the Spanish Inquisition, peppering the new hire with questions about their family, their old job, etc. Strike a balance between asking and sharing, allowing the new hire to engage at whatever level they are comfortable. Some will be quiet. Others will be chatty. Everyone is different. If a lunch or something similar isn't an option, consider having the new hire shadow a team member or receive an introductory level training from a co-worker. Early interaction with colleagues will accelerate their acclimation into the position.

While you want to provide a structured first day, you don't want the employee to be overwhelmed. Balance time spent with the employee with some time alone to process everything they are absorbing. Giving them a chance to sit and review documents, log in to their respective email and software accounts, or complete a solo task are great ways to build in this kind of time.

Before the end of the day, reconnect with the employee to ask questions and check in. Review plans for the next day or the rest of the week. Make sure they know how to reach you in the event they have questions or concerns. Before adjourning, reiterate your enthusiasm for their arrival and your desire to support them as they take on this new role.

The First Three Months

Being new is stressful. Many new employees have to shift from being the go-to person at their old job to being entirely dependent on others. Being new means no longer knowing the ins and outs of the operation, who to call in the face of problems, and how to contribute day in and day out. New hires often describe feeling stupid, overwhelmed, and exhausted while making the transition into a new role. The time and resources we provide to support them in the first three months on the job are integral to helping them develop competence again.

A designated mentor can be a valuable resource for a new employee. This is someone on the team assigned to be a supportive guide for the new employee. Prior to the employee's arrival, identify an established team member to serve as mentor. He or she can take on training duties or simply be a go-to person for questions and support. The mentor does not have to have the same job title as the new hire. Select a team member for this role who is positive, engaged with their job and the organization, and who appears to enjoy their work. The employee with the longest service time does not necessarily make the best mentor. Meet with the chosen mentor in advance of the new hire's arrival to discuss their role. Mentoring new hires can be a great stretch assignment for an employee.

It is also a way to offer autonomy, challenge, and purpose for that individual.

Leaders also play a key role in ensuring that the new hire isn't constantly looking for something to do. Otherwise, the new hire gets conveyor belted from place to place. What does this look like? Consider this story, shared by a new employee from an orientation program I led a few years back:

> *People didn't seem to know what to do with me. My boss said 'Why don't you go shadow Jim in the back? You can learn how we process lab reports that come in.' When I got back there the lab supervisor said 'Jim is unloading supplies. Why don't you go sit with Janine out front? I'm sure she could use the help.' When I found Janine she asked if I could come back in an hour. When I went back to ask my boss what I should do next, she had left for a two-hour meeting.*

Coming to work each day knowing that others have to find something for them to do can damage the morale of an employee. It furthers feelings of helplessness and frustration that come with being new. Thoughtful planning of the first few weeks on the job cuts down on this significantly. This takes time and effort on the part of the leader, but it is a key part of nurturing an employee's sense of importance right away.

As the months unfold begin to implement the strengths-based management approach outlined in Chapter 2. Identify the talents and skills of the individual and find ways for them to deploy their strengths on the job. Ask them to identify tasks or circumstances that energize them or that come easily and arrange for continued opportunities to do that work. This focus on strengths should start in the earliest stages of a new employee's tenure.

Make sure you set aside extra time to connect with the employee, review what they are learning, answer questions, and provide support. Cycle back to some of the information they received early on, including the job description and benefits information. It's foolhardy to believe that people hear something one time (and all at once) and retain it. Plan to revisit things more than once.

Experts suggest it takes six months to a year to become competent in a new job. Be patient. If the new employee is struggling, take a hard look at what did and did not take place during onboarding to determine if their struggles are related to performance or preparation.

Lastly, retain the notes, schedules, and materials you developed to onboard your new hire. You will likely need to orient new personnel again at some point. Don't reinvent the wheel. Use these materials to structure an intentional, well-planned onboarding process that can be used for all new hires. This will cut down on the time and effort it takes to welcome new members to the team.

WHAT PHYSICIANS AND MANAGERS MUST DO TO HIRE AND ONBOARD INTENTIONALLY

Action Items Summary:
- Don't rush through the selection process. Finding the right person takes time.

- Identify skills and behaviors needed for your open position. Craft behavioral-based interview questions that draw out a candidate's worthiness for a position.

- Be honest with candidates about the work environment and challenges they will face in the role.

- Call new hires to express enthusiasm and share important first day information.

- Announce the new hire to your team before their arrival. Ask for their help with welcoming and onboarding.

- Prepare a schedule for the new hire's first two weeks.

- Ensure the new employee's work station is clean and ready.

- Involve team members in the onboarding process.

- Give new hires a tour, job description, and clear purpose on the first day.

- Set two or three learning goals for the first two weeks on the job.

- Find ways to encourage interaction between the new hire and the rest of the team. Consider taking them to lunch with others.

- Assign the new hire a mentor.

- Set aside time to meet with and be available to the new hire in the first few weeks.

- Look for talents and strengths in the new employee. Put them to use as soon as possible.

- Continually check-in, encourage, and converse with the new employee.

- Retain onboarding materials for future new hires.

Chapter 8

You Must Continuously Share The Information Employees Need To Do Their Jobs

Carla was frustrated. A veteran operations manager overseeing four women's health clinics, she asked me to meet with her to discuss persistent staff issues. Sitting in a staff break room, I listened intently as she detailed many of the ways her team members continued to defy basic policies and expectations.

"I keep having the same conversations over and over," she said. "Like with lunch breaks. I've told the girls out front they can't break together because we don't have enough coverage to allow for it. But again and again I come in and here they are, sitting together, eating lunch at the same time. There are two girls in particular that just don't seem to get it."

"Take me through how you address that in the moment," I requested.

"I'll tell them that one of the girls needs to go back out front and that they can't eat together," she replied.

"How many times have you had that conversation in the past three months?" I asked.

"At least four, I'd say."

"What consequence have they experienced for continuing to do something that is not permitted?" I asked.

"Well, I keep having to talk to them about it."

We'll come back to that in a moment, I thought. "Are they aware of what the expectation is in those situations and why that expectation is in place?"

"Yes. I went over the policy in detail at a staff meeting. It was printed on their agenda and everything."

"How long ago was that?" I asked.

She thought for a moment then answered. "About two years ago," she said matter-of-factly.

• • • •

It is easy to assume malice. That underperforming employees aren't meeting expectations because they are lazy, uninvested, or simply don't care. While there are certainly times when this is the case, too often the problem lies with the leader and their failure to review and reinforce expectations as necessary.

In Carla's case, several issues were clearly present. First, team members were being expected to recall and act on a conversation that took place once in the distant past and not again since then. Second, the absence of a consequence for not changing their behavior meant the staff members in question were never given proof that the new behavior was a black-and-white expectation.

Yes, in a perfect world we would tell team members what they are expected to do, and then they would do it, without ever having to revisit the topic again. But how realistic is that? Think back to a meeting you participated in two years ago. Are the things discussed there ever-present in your mind? What about information you received six months ago? Probably not. We get distracted by what we must deal with day-to-day. Information and expectations fade from memory. We fall back into established routines of thinking and doing because they are established and routine. This happens not because we are lazy or uninvested or don't care, but because we are human.

The best leaders are teachers. And teaching is not a one-time event. Strong supervisors recognize that they must be the catalyst for continual review and reinforcement of the information employees need to succeed in their jobs.

That's not to let Carla's employees off the hook. They were clearly being insubordinate. However it's probable that, had Carla reviewed details about the expectation more frequently and initiated a consequence when presented with continued failure to comply, she likely would not have been having the same conversation repeatedly.

Expectations and consequences are just two examples of the types of information employees must hear, see, and internalize in order to perform in the ways leaders desire. They must be privy to updates and happenings related to their work environment. They need to periodically revisit processes, protocols, expectations, and policies to ensure comprehension and compliance. They need ongoing training in skills necessary to perform the job, ongoing feedback related to that performance, and tangible consequences when that performance isn't meeting expectations. And they need their leaders to model the very behaviors they are expected to exhibit.

Information leads to empowerment. Where teams lack a steady flow of important information, mistrust creeps in, gossip reigns, and engagement fades. This chapter outlines multiple actions physicians and managers must take to facilitate engagement through communication.

REVIEW AND REINFORCE

If you want employees to be invested in the success of your site, they must have exposure to most of the information you have as a leader. As a physician or manager, you see the big picture in ways employees often cannot. You participate in meetings and attend to operational details related to the health and stability of your site. You are tuned in to the politics and personalities that influence decision making and stand in the way of change. When you can't influence or aren't aware of what the future holds, at the very least you know that your power to act is limited.

Employee engagement depends on team members being in the know. Keep them informed about the financial health of your site. Provide updates about census and volume targets and whether they are being met. Clue them in to the reports, paperwork, projects, and compliance issues you tackle in your leadership role. They need to know about hiring, expansion, regulatory changes, billing issues, staffing and scheduling concerns, and anything else that influences the work you and they do.

One of the best physician leaders I ever worked with told me once, "I want people to make better decisions than I would make. That's why they need to know everything."

Employees with access to this kind of information are able to see the big picture. As a result, they make better decisions, are more tolerant of circumstances that prove challenging, and contribute in ways that transcend the tasks and responsibilities in their job description. Physicians and managers who want their personnel to act in this way must openly share information with their teams.

Learn, Do, and See

Think back to your days in elementary school. There's not a person reading this book who didn't participate in fire drills year after year after year. In fact, many of us still practice what to do in the event of a fire based on where we work. This is because repetition is key to learning. Fire drills allowed us to revisit the behavior expected in a particular situation and then practice it, so we knew exactly what to do and where to go if such a situation occurred. How we perform in almost any situation is determined by prior knowledge we had (what we learned), getting the chance to practice what is expected (what we do), and by observing those around us doing what is expected (what we see).

Leaders can impact performance with the same approach. Employee performance is shaped and improved by regularly reviewing scenarios, protocols, and policies, and through ongoing training. What does this look like? Set time aside to review service recovery steps and communicate your expectations for how to deal with agitated patients, and watch your team develop a higher level of skill and comfort in this area. Periodically revisit how to request supplies, process lab reports, or execute specific tasks in the electronic health record, for example, to keep processes uniform, reduce errors, and instill confidence in individual employees. Expose team members to recurrent training in skill areas related to their job like conflict resolution, software systems, and communication to keep those skills fresh. Successful leaders don't take these steps because they believe their staff lacks knowledge or is underperforming. They do it so team members can function with more autonomy and under less stress.

Another benefit to this kind of continuous review and reinforcement is that your team will need you to step in less frequently. Instead of being asked to clarify how to do something or intervene and do it for them, employees are instead able to execute because what to do is top of mind. And when your team doesn't have to come ask questions, you suddenly have more time to do those things that only you can do.

Facilitating learning for your team in this way doesn't have to take a lot of time. Spend ten minutes breaking down a case study or scenario at an upcoming staff meeting. If you hold quick huddles with your team, make a point to insert a reminder or two that reinforces steps in a process. Offer up an occasional email to your team with "helpful hints" or post them on a bulletin board in the staff lounge. For a structured way to plan and execute ongoing learning for your team, see the Resource Box in this chapter.

How to Create and Implement a Learning Calendar for your Team

1. **Identify 12 topics**. Think about everything team members need to know and act on: office procedures, computer systems, patient care protocols, staff expectations, communication and customer service, etc. These don't have to be problem areas or things staff only do infrequently. It's all about keeping important stuff fresh. Ask staff members, colleagues, and other stakeholders for suggestions.

2. **Assign one topic per month**. List January through December on a single sheet of paper and assign a subject to each month. It can be helpful to stagger areas of focus. For example: review something technical one month, a soft skill the next month, etc.

3. **Determine delivery mechanism**. Think about the best time and place to review the topic. As noted in this chapter, staff meetings and team huddles work well. Email can work too, but it's best for simple topics, as it doesn't allow for discussion. Here again an annual or bi-annual staff retreat is a great option. Don't shy away from scheduling a standalone training from time to time either.

4. **Identify and invite reviewers.** Who is best equipped to visit (or revisit) the material with the team? Identify a subject matter expert for your topic. It can be you, another leader, a staff member, or an authority on the subject from outside your organization. Invite them to take the lead on the topic as scheduled.

5. **Finalize and share.** Once all the details are finalized, put all the information into a single page document. Share it with the other managers and physicians on site to get support and buy-in. Once everyone has seen it, share it with your team, along with your reasons for developing the plan.

Be a Role Model

Employees receive information every day in another way that shapes their behavior and performance on the job. It comes in the form of the observed behavior of those around them. Remember the statistics on adult learning from Chapter 5? Research suggests we retain 10% of what we read, 15% of what we hear, and 85% of what we observe. This is why the daily presence of strong role models shapes employee performance in a positive way. Research shows that leaders who establish norms for team behavior and then personally model the norms get higher levels of engagement from their teams.

Conversely, if toxic team members are present or there are leaders with bad habits, then the wrong kinds of messages get sent, reinforced, and over time become a part of the culture. Take a close look at the voices that wield influence over your team. Do they set an example for others? Do they send mixed messages by not fulfilling the very expectations of the team? Be sure to look in the mirror as well. Do you practice what you preach?

Unfortunately, I've worked with many leaders who face this challenging scenario: They expect staff to conduct themselves in a certain way, yet someone is present whose behavior sabotages the culture you are trying to create. Sometimes it is a direct report. Other times it is a physician. In most cases, a frank conversation is necessary. It can be intimidating to approach a colleague or superior to ask them to alter their behavior. In almost every case though, the truth works well. Be prepared to directly and concisely describe the issue at hand and the ways that it negatively impacts the team and site. If you are tuned into what matters most to the person you are speaking with, align your concerns with those outcomes. For example, if you need to speak with a physician who is known to place a priority on optimized patient flow, try to connect the behavior you are concerned about with that issue (Ex. "When you raise your voice to the staff it rattles them, slowing everything down."). Ensure that any attempt you make to have such a conversation is heavy on courtesy and respect.

This is but one example of when it is necessary for you to find the leadership courage to initiate a feedback conversation. Feedback, it turns out, and your ability to share it clearly and often, plays a large role in determining the engagement levels of your team.

FEEDBACK

Ask any leader what comes to mind when they hear the word "feedback" and they are likely to give similar answers. Constructive criticism. Ways to improve. Addressing problematic behavior. While these answers certainly belong in a conversation about the subject, feedback is much more than just comments and suggestions. Feedback refers to *all* the ways – positive, constructive, and purposeful - leaders share information that shapes performance and engages employees.

If you are like most leaders then you received little in the way of formal training for feedback conversations. It is somewhat remarkable that we hire and promote people into management positions, most of which require that person to address or shape employee performance through dialogue, yet we rarely prepare or measure for the ability. Have you ever been on a job interview where you were asked to demonstrate giving performance feedback? I haven't. You probably haven't either.

But feedback isn't just something you *should* do. It is something you *must* do. It is one of the fundamental obligations that comes with being a leader.

The Job Is Feedback

Early in my career, over lunch with a friend, I was bemoaning having to address a concern I had about an employee's behavior. I hated having to spend energy figuring out how to communicate my concerns. I was angry that the employee had put me in the position to experience the anxiety and stress I felt in the face of an uncomfortable conversation. After a few minutes of what was clearly whining, my friend, who was also a colleague, said something to me that's stayed with me since then.

"Oh for goodness' sake, Joe...get over it. It's your job."

I felt like I had been slapped awake. I had long hated the performance feedback conversations I had to have in my role. They made me nervous and uncomfortable. I wanted no part of them and grew frustrated when it became obvious I had to have one. In that moment I realized I had been trying to figure out how to eliminate them from my job, rather than focusing on how to get better at having them. Her comment crystalized something for me that has remained since: If I want to serve in a leadership role I *have* to give feedback. That's what the job *is*.

For any leader, feedback is an *obligation*.

Why? Because feedback is central to most everything a leader hopes to accomplish. It is a crucial part of helping employees understand their impact, connect to a larger purpose, and experience recognition. And yes, it's how we address poor or inappropriate performance, but also how leaders propel employees' abilities and contributions to another level.

Feedback isn't just the addressing of performance concerns. When physicians and managers explain a different way to complete a step in a process or talk with an employee about altering their interactions with a patient, they are giving feedback. When they pull a team member aside to thank them for making a difference that day, they are giving feedback. When leaders tell any of the four *purpose* stories outlined in Chapter 6, they are giving feedback. Annual performance reviews, one-on-one meetings, and dialogue between co-workers are all important delivery systems for feedback and all contribute to creating the conditions that lead to engagement. (Do you struggle with those annual performance evaluations? Yet another great resource included in the free *Cure for the Common Leader* Resource Kit is a free guide to *Performance Reviews that Get Results*. Head over to <u>CureForTheCommonLeader.com</u> to download the kit now.*)*

In each chapter of this book I've outlined an abundance of information that employees need to hear from physicians and managers. Their talents and strengths. That their opinions and ideas are valued. How to progress on their desired career path. How to navigate conflict on the team. The impact of their work. It was stated in Chapter 2 that one-on-one meetings are the lifeblood of employee engagement. Why? Because they are where you hear from and talk to employees. One-on-ones provide a continuous opportunity to give all kinds of feedback. Indeed, you have an obligation to do just that, otherwise you will never accomplish what you were hired to do.

Some feedback conversations can be tough. At times you will tell someone something they don't want to hear or don't agree with. You will have no choice but to live in the discomfort of another person's anger because to not do so would mean not giving them the information they need to *do their job*. For that reason, and because it is such an area of discomfort for so many, let's explore a brief primer on giving feedback to address performance concerns.

Giving Performance Feedback

The key to giving performance feedback is differentiating between descriptive language and behavioral language. Descriptive language is heavy on adjectives that have meaning for the speaker but lack clarity for the employee. Behavioral language pinpoints the specific, observable actions leaders want employees to stop or start taking. Unfortunately many who initiate feedback conversations tend to use descriptive language heavily. Informing someone they need to *try harder, be more organized,* or *stop being negative* is vague and subjective. It also lays a values judgment upon the employee that is received as a character flaw, which leads to defensiveness, outrage, or "shutting down."

Focusing on behaviors means describing the actions the employee did or did not take. Prior to the feedback conversation identify what you want the employee to do differently. Be prepared to cite specific examples or events. For instance, instead of advising an employee that they need to be *friendlier* to patients, say instead, *"You need to smile, make eye contact, and display more energy when greeting patients."* Not only do you provide the receiver with clear instructions on how to improve, they are less likely to experience this feedback as critical of *them*.

It sounds fairly straightforward, but after years of training leaders in this area, I can tell you it takes practice. Once you begin intentionally using behavioral language, the quality and results of your feedback conversations will improve dramatically. Other keys to delivering feedback effectively:

- **Prepare.** Take time to identify the behavior change that needs to occur. Make sure you have specific examples to highlight. Consider role playing with a colleague or supervisor to get ready for a tough talk.

- **Be direct and concise**. Know what you want to say, say it, and then be quiet. Stay out of your own way. If there's silence, resist the urge to fill it. They will. And that's often where insight lives.

- **Be specific and objective**. Avoid generalities like *everyone, never,* and *always*. Identify specific events, behaviors, outcomes, or conversations.

- **Include cause and effect.** *"When _____ happens it results in _____."* Make a case for why the concern you are expressing should concern them.

- **Address behavior, not personality**. Remember, behavior is observable and documentable. It's something you can watch someone do. Differentiate between performance that needs to improve and quirks of personality that, while perhaps annoying, are not appropriate for supervisor intervention.

- **Don't be freaked if feelings show up**. The person you are speaking to is a human being. We emote. Don't get rattled if it happens. It's part of the gig. Pause a moment for dignity then talk through it respectfully.

- **Be specific about expectations going forward**. Discuss the change you are looking for. Ask for that change. If speaking with a direct report you may be able to mandate. Giving feedback laterally (to a colleague) or up (to a superior) will require coming to agreement on future steps through dialogue.

- **Don't apologize** for giving feedback. Starting off with, "I'm sorry to have to tell you this…" is like saying, "I'm sorry for having this thought but I'm going to say it anyway."

- **Don't ask, "How are you feeling?"** This focuses on their emotional response to getting feedback rather than on the substance of what was said. Instead ask, "What are your thoughts?"

- **Use open-ended questions**. Ask, "How do you think we should proceed?" "What steps can we take to change this?" Open-ended questions invite discussion responses. Avoid Yes/No questions ("Do you think you can make that change?" "Do you understand?"). You get one-word answers ("Yes.") and no proof.

- **Be the calmest person in the room.** If they escalate, avoid matching them. Call for a break or reschedule if emotions are running high.

- **Discuss.** Feedback isn't a one-way street. Be prepared to engage in a dialogue about what you shared. Be open to their input. Treat it as new information to consider.

- **Ask them to restate what they heard.** Try saying, "I want to make sure I've done a good job explaining my concern. Can you repeat back to me what you heard?" This brings clarity to the feedback and cuts down on the employee hyperbolizing your concerns afterwards.

- **Follow-up.** Document what was agreed upon. Take time to discuss the feedback again shortly after the initial conversation. Point out the positive impact of any changed behavior.

From Words to Action

For many employees, being told that behavior change is necessary isn't enough. If you've taken steps to articulate the specific changes needed and the reasons why change is necessary, yet no change ensues, you may need to enact consequences for failure to change.

Psychologists suggest that three conditions must be present to facilitate behavior change. First, the person needs to see a benefit to the change. Second, they need to believe they are capable of making the change. This is referred to as self-efficacy. Third, there must be a consequence for not changing. Often change occurs only when the pain of staying the same finally outweighs the pain of the change. For leaders, this means initiating consequences when the requested change does not appear in the aftermath of feedback conversations.

Many organizations, especially those with human resources departments, have formal corrective action steps that leaders must follow. These may include documentation of a formal verbal warning, a written warning, a probation period, or a structured performance improvement agreement, among others. In most cases these steps culminate in some kind of final warning. If improvement does not occur in the aftermath of these steps, termination becomes necessary.

It's not uncommon to encounter front-line leaders who are hesitant to enact formal steps when employees do not amend performance in the ways requested by the boss. This occurs for numerous reasons:

fear of conflict, ambiguity in how to proceed, not wanting to be the "bad guy," and more. But failing to act in these circumstances enables the employee to continue with the undesirable behavior because they have not yet experienced all the conditions necessary to prompt change. A lack of consequences for poor or inappropriate performance also damages team morale. There is a cost to both culture and team performance when some on the team are allowed to "coast" or get away with not meeting expectations.

If one or two feedback conversations have taken place, yet no change is imminent, it's time to take stronger action. Identify appropriate next steps and get buy-in from business partners, including human resources and other members of your leadership team. Set up a time to present the consequences to the employee and reiterate the new behavior that is expected. Set a deadline by which the change must occur and outline what will happen if the employee fails to comply. Document the conversation in a formal letter or via email. There are only two paths for supervisors in these situations. The employee either improves or is separated from the position.

As a leader of people, you will never get away from having to face some tough conversations. You will always have to talk with people who are underperforming. Great leaders take an empathetic view. Never forget that every single person that works for you is a fully formed human being. They are somebody's mother, or sister, or son. They face struggles and pressures and stresses that you don't know about and that they aren't obligated to share. Address the workplace behavior that needs to change without making a values judgment on the person. Bring your compassion to these interactions and don't assume malice on the part of the employee until they give you evidence of malice. Above all else, never belittle or dismiss someone's worth simply because they aren't working out on the job. Everyone has a right to courtesy, dignity, and respect.

Performance feedback conversations can be challenging. So, too, can the additional steps leaders must take to hold employees to account. Your employees might react strongly. It's not easy to be the target of someone's anger or dislike. It's not easy to know they are vilifying you to others in the office or to friends and family over dinner. But it is your job. If you've been managing others for some time, you have probably already had conversations that resulted in anger or disagreement or discomfort. Let's accept that, from time to time, it's one of the necessary evils of being in a leadership role. Or, as my friend so eloquently put it a few years ago: "Get over it. It's your job."

WHAT PHYSICIANS AND MANAGERS MUST DO TO CONTINUOUSLY SHARE INFORMATION

Action Items Summary:

- Don't assume malice. Identify the information employees need to buy-in and perform.

- Use staff meetings, team huddles, one-on-ones, email, and on-site posting to share information.

- Revisit processes, protocols, and expectations continuously.

- Consider drafting an annual learning calendar for your team.

- Provide access to additional training and continuing education to further skills and keep them fresh.

- Model the behavior you expect from team members. Address those who undermine or compromise the performance expected of others.

- Accept that giving feedback is a fundamental part of the job of a leader.

- Focus on specific behaviors during feedback conversations. Avoid descriptive language, as it is vague and subjective.

- Failure to change must come with consequences. Move employees through a formal corrective action process when feedback fails to prompt change.

Chapter 9
Putting It All Together

Success in healthcare is determined first and foremost by the care delivered to patients and families and the quality of the interactions they have across all aspects of their healthcare experience. While leaders at all levels must manage a variety of technical and task-related responsibilities, it is the shaping of the environment, relationships, and experiences of employees to create engagement that leads to the ideal patient experience. Simply executing a handful of ideas from this book can have an impact, but it won't be enough to create lasting change. Engaged, motivated employees are the result of thoughtfully creating the conditions employees need to be at their best and meticulously attending to them over the long term. This requires a commitment to an overall engagement philosophy. Because employee engagement is not a destination, it is a journey.

Work environments are built on daily routines of thinking and doing. With planning and intentionality, the actions advocated for in the chapters of this book can transform your environment into one that contains everything employees need to give their all and be at their best. This chapter will help you apply all you have learned.

START WITH A LEADERSHIP PARTNERSHIP

The manager-physician relationship can be a challenging dynamic. Physicians have unique goals, difficulties, concerns, and needs. Managers, too, have a host of challenges and responsibilities exclusive to their role. What must be understood by both parties is that the environment employees need to become psychologically committed to their work can only be created when physicians and managers develop and share a collaborative leadership partnership. This is truly the first step on a journey to engagement.

Physicians and managers must recognize and respect the role their counterparts have in running a successful clinical site. Where a leadership partnership is absent, engagement suffers and people management challenges appear. When the staff doesn't like something they hear from one leader, they run to the other. When mistrust between leaders is present, communication, decision making, and change management become exponentially difficult. To form and maintain a successful leadership partnership, physicians and managers must first understand where the other is coming from.

Managers need to remember that when it comes to physicians, it's their name on the door. For that reason, they desire ownership of and influence over every aspect of care delivery. The volume of patients, wait times, and patient flow are tied directly to the doctor. They believe that, above all else, their daily performance, clinical expertise, and the ability of the staff to support their efforts determines the success and effectiveness of the clinical site. Their first priority is to evaluate, diagnose, and treat patients as efficiently and completely as possible. Everything else comes second. Every day they go to work and take the lives and livelihoods of others into their hands. If something goes wrong, the doctor is the one who gets sued. It is the doctor's name that gets reported and publicized. For these reasons, they want to be heard and made aware of everything going on in the practice.

Physicians need to remember that when it comes to operations managers, it's their name on the org chart. They are the direct supervisor for the personnel in the office. To be effective, they need to be empowered by the physicians to make decisions and lead others. In addition to coordinating schedules, staffing, and numerous processes, they must navigate and attend to the emotions and personalities of those on the team. Managers know their docs want them to run a well-oiled machine without excuses. What they require to do so successfully is trust in their judgment. And while the physician's name and reputation are on the line every day, if something goes wrong it is the manager who likely receives the first phone call. They will be asked to verify that institutional policies were followed, staff completed required training, and that all appropriate documentation is in order. The manager will be expected to assist any investigation, testify if legal action results, and in most states can be terminated at will (operations managers don't have employment or incentive contracts). For these reasons, they need authority, credibility, and respect from all on the team, most especially the physicians.

Clearly, both have a lot at stake. A successful leadership partnership requires mutual respect, trust, and ongoing communication. Meet frequently to shape that partnership. Discuss ongoing challenges and share information, ideas, and opinions. Agree to present a united front to the team at all times, and know what kinds of issues the other prefers to take the lead on. For example, the physicians may ask the manager to defer all clinical, procedural, and patient care issues to them. The manager in turn may ask that all scheduling, staffing, organizational policy, and team interpersonal issues be steered their way. Disagree in private and work to avoid the intrusion of ego. Back each other up. Involve other supervisors and clinicians on the team with management responsibilities as appropriate, with everything flowing up to the leadership partnership.

Because both physicians and managers are bosses in the eyes of the team, both must take an active role in meeting the workplace needs of employees. A leadership partnership between managers and physicians can be a fulfilling and powerful one in a healthcare setting. It won't develop without the investment of time and trust, and it won't happen overnight.

PUTTING THIS BOOK INTO ACTION

My hope is that by the time you have reached this final chapter your mind is percolating with ideas on how to foster engagement on your team. While you may be tempted to dive right in, you will be far more successful if your efforts are calculated. The first step of a planned approach is to invite a critical mass of leaders on your team to read this book then move collectively through the *diagnosis, action planning*, and *implementation* steps outlined below. Doing so increases your chances of a well-thought-out enactment of the material presented here. Or consider forming an engagement team for this purpose that includes employees. If you are alone in your efforts to improve the performance of your team, the steps outlined below are still appropriate and will help you plan and execute a targeted approach.

Diagnosis

Begin by evaluating which of the seven habits outlined in this book you do well or are already displayed with frequency at your site. This is probably obvious to you already. The most thorough diagnostic approach is to revisit the Action Items Summary at the end of each chapter and put a check mark next to each suggestion that is currently not in place or not happening at your site. The chapter with the most checkmarks will be your greatest area of need, and so on, and so on. I encourage leadership teams to do this from an overall environmental perspective, but also that individual leaders do this to account for their own areas of focus or improvement.

As your engagement team (or you as an individual) moves through this process, it's also important to evaluate engagement at the employee level. Survey your employees to evaluate what they experience and what is missing. With this book as the premise, the 10 questions below can serve as a basic employee engagement survey. They should be presented in the form of statements with respondents rating their level of agreement on a Likert Scale (Strongly Agree, Agree, Neutral, Disagree, and Strongly Disagree):

1. I get to use my talents and strengths in my day-to-day work.

2. My colleagues and supervisors care about me as a person.

3. At work, my ideas and opinions are solicited and considered.

4. I have opportunities at work to form friendly relationships with my teammates.

5. Leadership keeps me up to date on what's happening in the organization.

6. I have the materials, equipment, and resources necessary to do my job effectively.

7. I regularly receive feedback about my work.

8. The training I received when I arrived adequately prepared me for my job.

9. In my role I am given opportunities to learn and grow.

10. I do important work that makes a difference.

Allow employees to complete the survey anonymously and compile the results. Note that surveying employees sets up an expectation of action. Research has shown that inaction in the aftermath of employee engagement surveys leads to disengagement. Be prepared to take demonstrative action within a reasonable time frame of surveying your team.

Action Planning

Once you've identified your greatest areas of need, begin identifying the actionable items suggested in this book to enact the associated engagement strategies. For example, if your analysis of your environment points to a lack of adequate training during new hire orientation, and this is echoed in the survey results you receive from employees, revisit that chapter in this book and identify the actions you will take to begin addressing this deficiency. If your diagnostic efforts indicate that you need to implement most or all of what is discussed in this book, prioritize your greatest areas of need.

If you are unsure of where to begin I recommend starting with purpose. Do the work outlined in Chapter 6 (You Must Connect Each Employee To A Powerful Purpose) right away. Showing employees the impact they have can benefit any team at any level of engagement. The other action I suggest you take right away is to begin holding one-on-one meetings with direct reports. As outlined in Chapter 2 (You Must Manage Individually) these serve as a crucial delivery system for many of the conditions employees must experience to thrive. Still not sure where to start? For a list of simple strategies you can begin using right now, without delay, check out the Resource Box in this chapter.

Effective action plans are time and date specific. Once you have identified the actions needed to address your greatest areas of need, commit to their implementation over a two- to three- month period. Don't try to do too much too quickly. This may overwhelm staff or be perceived as disingenuous. Construct an implementation calendar with tasks, meetings, topics, and events scheduled as appropriate. Make this a six-month calendar and plan the second wave of implementation that will follow your initial efforts. Be sure to include regular meetings of your leadership or engagement team (if you aren't flying solo) to review and revise your plan as needed.

15 Actions that Motivate & Engage

Motivation and engagement come from the continuous tiny actions, conversations, and reminders leaders deploy daily. Here are 15 actions to motivate and engage that take less than 15 minutes a day.

1. Ask someone for their opinion on a problem you are facing. ("How would you..." or "What would you recommend?")

2. Mention an upcoming training opportunity.

3. Give voice to someone's contribution.

4. Share an impact story that reinforces purpose.

5. Ask about someone's weekend/holiday/leisure plans.

6. Point out a team member's unique talent or skill.

7. Ask, "What energizes you about your job? Why?"

8. Take an inventory of the materials and equipment being used. What can you upgrade?

9. Share someone's contribution/effort/accomplishment with *your* boss.

10. Call a new hire to check in and share your excitement about their impending arrival.

11. Offer to do a task others dread.

12. Invite someone to partner with you on an upcoming task or project.

13. Point out an improvement someone has made.

14. Remind someone why their work is so important.

15. Ask someone what they'd like to try and do that they've never done before.

Implementation

At this point you are aware of your needs and the actions necessary to address them. You (perhaps along with others) have crafted a time-specific plan for implementation. Well done. Now...begin!

As you execute your action plan, tell your staff what you are doing and why. Be honest with them (I'm sure you read that in this book somewhere!). There is no shame in telling your team that you are making an effort to improve their work experience and grow as a leader. Most will find this admirable. As you attempt to install the conditions that lead to engagement, keep these behaviors at the fore:

- **Give feedback**: Provide feedback to staff on the quality of their work and their interactions with patients. Identify ways for them to improve. Sing their praises when they demonstrate desired behaviors. Pull them aside when they're underperforming. Help debrief staff after a difficult interaction. Talk through alternative approaches and solutions. Provide a balance of challenge and support as needed. Remember the old adage: Praise loudly, criticize gently.

- **Be a Role Model**: Leaders work in a fishbowl. Every action taken (or not) and every word spoken (or not) shapes the culture of the workplace. Show up every day with the attitude, energy, and approach you ask for from others. Demonstrate ideal interactions with patients and family members, colleagues and subordinates. Admit your mistakes. Be an example to others of how to treat people and do good work.

- **Communicate, communicate, communicate**: Give voice to the mission, vision, and values of your organization and the powerful purpose at the centerpiece of everything employees do. Help those you lead to connect the dots between that purpose and their individual work. Help them see the ways that the seemingly inconsequential parts of their job impact others. Provide ongoing updates in team huddles, staff meetings, and one-on-ones with members of your team.

- **Recognize**: Find ways to recognize staff individually and collectively. Praise specific ways they serve patients, help colleagues, or make a difference to the team. Say "thank you" often. Recognition from an on-site leader has been shown to be a more powerful workplace motivator than money and perks. A small dose of recognition can have a large impact.

Implementation must also include ongoing evaluation. Periodically benchmark your efforts against the behaviors advocated for in this book. Re-survey your team six months after your initial action plan implementation, then annually thereafter. Examine the key performance indicators and metrics that your organization uses to define health and stability including turnover, retention, patient complaints, new and repeat visits, and revenue. If problem areas exist in these metrics determine if elements of disengagement are contributing and where. Commit to fostering a culture of engagement by discussing engagement elements at weekly meetings, planning sessions, and in one-on-one meetings.

CONCLUSION

By now it should be obvious that the most engaged and inspired healthcare teams don't get that way through happenstance. Multiple forces conspire to shape the environment that employees travel to for work each day but none is more powerful than the physicians and managers they call "boss." While it takes time and energy to create the conditions that lead to engagement, it doesn't take much at all to create disengagement. It really is a fragile thing. Just one uninvested manager, one bullying physician, or one toxic contributor can upend it all. That's why leaders must commit to fostering a culture of engagement and work daily to sustain it. When this effort is continually present engagement feeds itself and becomes easier to sustain over time.

The good news is that engaging and inspiring your healthcare teams does not require you to scrape for resources or build a new budget. There is almost no monetary cost associated with executing the habits described in this book. Truly, the most significant expense is time. Thankfully many of the recommendations made herein require just a modicum of time. Most of what I've shared with you can be added to your daily routine with little disruption. For those recommendations that do take time, isn't it worth it? How much time would you trade to stack your team with engaged and inspired contributors who put forth maximum effort and are genuinely invested in your overall success?

Employees don't become engaged overnight. Time, commitment, and perseverance are your best weapons against lagging engagement over the course of employees' tenure. Don't be overwhelmed by all that we've discussed. The answer to the question "How do I motivate people" is not a complex one. Invest in and involve your employees from the day they arrive. Manage them as individuals and care about them as people. Give them a chance to connect with each other and to a powerful purpose. Provide the information they need to do their jobs. Hold people accountable and remove toxic contributors. Solicit their ideas. Celebrate their contributions. Meet with them, support them, and encourage them to learn and grow. It really is that simple.

My favorite definition of leadership is a simple one: Leadership is creating the conditions necessary for people to thrive. You now know what those conditions are. You now know the actions you must take. In the high-stress, compassion-demanding environment that is healthcare, it's up to you to give your employees what they need to thrive. Your team needs you to do it. The patients and families they see every day need you to do it.

After all, if you don't do it...who will?

Acknowledgements

Ask anyone who has written a book and they will tell you it does not happen without a lot of help. To my amazing (big!) family, thank you for your unending love and support. To Renee and Kathy, my fellow masterminders, the accountability, support, knowledge, and resources we've shared has been invaluable. I am so grateful to know and work with you both. Bonnie Budzowski, this book would not exist without you. You are a terrific coach and an even better person. Thank you for all your advice, wisdom, and support. Thanks also go to Henry DeVries and Mark LeBlanc for your coaching and your help with the title and to Weston Lyon and his team at Plug & Play Publishing. Thank you for getting me across the finish line.

There are so many healthcare professionals who contributed in one way or another to this book that it would be a daunting task to list them all by name, so please forgive this more generalized approach. To all the men and women who have generously given their time and attention to my workshops, seminars, retreats, keynotes, and breakouts, thank you for allowing me to do this work I love so much and for the enthusiasm you continue to show for it. To all the members of my Elite Healthcare Managers Coaching & Mastermind Group and my individual coaching clients: I learn from you every day and am humbled and honored to be a part of your professional development. A special thanks goes to Jim and Nadine at ACMS for the faith you showed in me and in Ally Training & Development from its earliest days. And of course, to the amazing managers and providers who so generously gave interviews specifically for this book, thank you for sharing your stories, headaches, time, and insight. I couldn't have done it without you.

Above all others I send my greatest thanks to Jess, Lily, and Miles. You are the reason for everything.

Resources and References

The following publications contributed to the content of this book:

BOOKS

Drive: The Surprising Truth About What Motivates Us by Daniel Pink

The Servant Leader by John Stahl-Wert and Ken Jennings

Strengths Based Leadership by T. Rath and B. Conchie

StrengthsFinder 2.0 by Tom Rath

Understanding and Changing Your Management Style by Robert Benfari

Encouraging the Heart by James Kouzes and Barry Posner

Leading Change by John Kotter

Journey to the Emerald City by Roger Connors and Tom Smith

The 7 Habits of Highly Effective People by Steven Covey

Servant Leadership by Robert Greenleaf

Helping People Win at Work by Ken Blanchard and Garry Ridge

The Interprofessional Healthcare Team: Leadership and Development by Donna Weiss, Felice Tilin, and Marlene Morgan

Gifts Differing: Understanding Personality Type by Isabel Briggs-Myers with Peter B. Myers

ARTICLES and REPORTS

"The State of the American Workplace (2012 Report)" by Gallup, Gallup.com

"Strengths-Based Development in Practice" by Timothy D. Hodges and Donald O. Clifton, Positive Psychology in Practice (2004)

"Manager Meetings and Motivation," Zigarmi, Diehl, Houson, and Witt, *Training Magazine* (2013)

"Stages of Group Development," Bruce Tuckman (model published 1977)

"Positive Affect and the Complete Dynamics of Human Flourishing," Marciel Losada and Barbara Fredrickson, *American Psychologist* (2005)

"Developing Healthcare Leaders: What We Have Learned and What is Next," Garman and Lemak, National Center for Healthcare Leadership White Paper (2011)

"Addressing the Leadership Gap in Healthcare: What's Needed When it Comes to Leader Talent?" Center for Creative Leadership (2011)

"Leadership Development Curriculum for Chief Residents in Medicine," Accreditation Council for Graduate Medical Education, Council of Review Committee Residents (2012)

"Healthcare Leadership Competency Model (v2.1)," National Center for Healthcare Leadership, Copyright 2006, All Rights Reserved.

"Occupational Outlook Handbook 2013-2014," U.S. Bureau of Labor Statistics, www.bls.gov

"A Theory of Human Motivation," A. Maslow, *Psychological Review* #50 (1943) p.370-396.

"The Employment Interview: A Review of Current Studies and Directions for Future Research," Macan, *Human Resource Management Review v19* (2009) p.203–218

"The Transtheoretical Model and Stages of Change," JO Prochaska, CA Redding, KE Evers (1977)

"Trends in Global Employee Engagement," AonHewitt (2014) www.aon.com

"Employee Engagement Research Report Update," BlessingWhite (2013) www.blessingwhite.com

"Employee Work Passion, Volume 7," Zigarmi, Houson, Diehl, and Witt. (2014) The Ken Blanchard Companies

Book Today and
Waive All Travel Expenses

Are there physicians and managers in your organization that don't know how to lead, develop, and motivate their teams?

Are you spending time and money on training with few results?

Would your leaders/members benefit from hearing much of the content covered in this book in a dynamic, time-sensitive workshop?

If you answered YES to any of these questions - visit CureForTheCommonLeader.com or contact Joe directly at joe@allytraining.com or 412-977-9928 - to have him come to your business or organization.

For a limited time, readers can book Joe **without paying travel expenses**!

Joe travels the country, visiting healthcare systems, medical societies, hospital associations, and professional organizations, teaching physicians and managers evidence-based ways to improve engagement and become better bosses.

In his keynotes and workshops, participants learn:
- What leaders must do to build teams that work hard, get along, and wow patients.

- How to transform employees into superstar contributors who care and try every single day.

- How to rehabilitate sleepwalkers and daydreamers who are doing the minimum or going through the motions.

- Ways to quickly, clearly, and comfortably address disruptive, inconsistent or toxic employee behavior.

- Critical soft-skills like giving feedback, coaching others, and teambuilding so they can stop managing sites and start leading people.

A dynamic speaker, Joe's audiences rave about his programs and keynotes:

"The BEST seminar I have ever attended. It reinforced info I already knew, taught me so much more, and gave me tools to be a better leader. I feel energized. This is material I will use for a lifetime." ~Cynthia Hirt, RN & Office Manager, Pittsburgh, PA

"Incredibly valuable. Joe's approach to training is personal and effective. I took away more specific and actionable items related to motivation and engagement than in week-long conferences." ~Amanda Hansen, Asst. Dir of Pharmacy, Cleveland Clinic

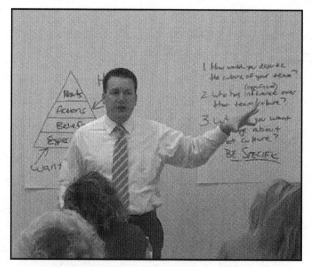

Joe Mull teaching a leadership masterclass
for physicians and managers.

"Even now, months after the training, we're still using this every day. You make every person want to be a better manager, role model, and employee after completing a training with you!" ~Kathy Aaron, Office Manager, Magee Women's Specialty Services, Franklin, PA

"Joe came highly recommended to us by several of our members. Besides facilitating a dynamic, impactful program, Joe also provided us everything we needed to market the event, including emails, flyers, etc. If you are looking for a low-stress way to provide 'value-added' experiences to your members, I encourage you to connect with Joe Mull." ~James Ireland, Asst. Executive Director, Allegheny County Medical Society, PA

Whether you book a keynote for a conference or a day-long masterclass for your managers and physicians, just mention you've read this book and Joe will ***waive all travel expenses for the booking!***

To get started, visit **CureForTheCommonLeader.com** or contact Joe directly at joe@allytraining.com or 412-977-9928.

Made in the USA
Middletown, DE
02 March 2016